ABDOMINAL PAIN

A GUIDE TO
RAPID DIAGNOSIS

D0070789

ABDOMINAL PAIN

A GUIDE TO
RAPID DIAGNOSIS

Lloyd M. Nyhus, MD, FACS
Warren H. Cole Professor of Surgery
Head Emeritus
Department of Surgery
University of Illinois College of Medicine at Chicago
Chicago, Illinois

Joseph M. Vitello, MD
Assistant Professor of Surgery
University of Illinois College of Medicine
Attending Surgeon
West Side Veterans Hospital
Chicago, Illinois

Robert E. Condon, MD, MS, FACS
Ausman Foundation Professor and Chairman
Department of Surgery
Medical College of Wisconsin
Chief of Staff
Froedtert Memorial Lutheran Hospital
Milwaukee, Wisconsin

APPLETON & LANGE
Norwalk, Connecticut

95 96 97 98 / 10 9 8 7 6 5 4 3 2 1

Prentice Hall International (UK) Limited, *London*
Prentice Hall of Australia Pty. Limited, *Sydney*
Prentice Hall Canada, Inc., *Toronto*
Prentice Hall Hispanoamericana, S. A., *Mexico*
Prentice Hall of India Private Limited, *New Delhi*
Prentice Hall of Japan, Inc., *Tokyo*
Simon & Schuster Asia Pte.. Ltd., *Singapore*
Editora Prentice Hall do Brasil Ltda., *Rio de Janeiro*
Prentice Hall, *Englewood Cliffs, New Jersey*

Library of Congress Cataloging-in-Publication Data
Nyhus, Lloyd M. (Lloyd Milton), 1923–
    Abdominal pain : a guide to rapid diagnosis / Lloyd M. Nyhus,
Joseph M. Vitello, Robert E. Condon.
        p. cm.
    ISBN 0-8385-0068-4
    1. Abdominal pain—Diagnosis. I. Vitello, Joseph M. II. Condon,
Robert E. (Robert Edward), 1929– . III. Title.
    [DNLM: 1. Abdominal Pain—diagnosis. WI 147 N994a 1994]
RC944.N94 1994
617.5'075—dc20
DNLM/DLC   94-21712
for Library of Congress   CIP

Acquisitions Editor: Jane Licht
Production Editor: Sondra Greenfield
Designer: Michael J. Kelly
Cover Design: Mary Skudlarek

ISBN 0-8385-0068-4

90000

9 780838 500682

PRINTED IN THE UNITED STATES OF AMERICA

Contents

v

Contributors

Charles Aprahamian, MD
Professor of Surgery
Medical College of Wisconsin
Chief, Section of Trauma and Emergency Surgery
Milwaukee Regional Medical Center
Milwaukee, Wisconsin

Christopher P. Brandt, MD
Assistant Professor of Surgery
Case Western Reserve University
Attending Surgeon
MetroHealth Medical Center
Cleveland, Ohio

Robert E. Condon, MD, MS, FACS
Ausman Foundation Professor and Chairman
Department of Surgery
Medical College of Wisconsin
Chief of Staff
Froedtert Memorial Lutheran Hospital
Milwaukee, Wisconsin

Bernardo Duarte, MD
Chief, Division of General Surgery
Veterans Administration West Side Center
Chicago, Illinois

Alfredo J. Fabrega, MD
Assistant Professor of Surgery
University of Illinois at Chicago
Transplant Surgeon
University of Illinois Hospital and Clinics
Chicago, Illinois

John Fildes, MD
Assistant Professor of Surgery
University of Illinois at Chicago
Division Chief, Trauma Education and Research
Cook County Hospital
Chicago, Illinois

Joseph Kokoszka
Resident in Surgery
University of Illinois Affiliated Hospitals
Chicago, Illinois

Mark A. Malangoni, MD
Professor and Vice Chairman, Department of Surgery
Case Western Reserve University
Chairperson, Department of Surgery
MetroHealth Medical Center
Cleveland, Ohio

Janet L. Meller, MD
Assistant Professor of Surgery
University of Chicago College of Medicine at Chicago
Attending Surgeon
University of Illinois Hospital
Chicago, Illinois

Lloyd M. Nyhus, MD, FACS
Warren H. Cole Professor of Surgery
Head Emeritus
Department of Surgery
University of Illinois College of Medicine at Chicago
Chicago, Illinois

Colathur K. Palani, MD, FACS
Clinical Associate Professor of Surgery
Loyola University
Maywood, Illinois
Associate Academic Director of Surgery
MacNeal Hospital
Berwyn, Illinois

Raymond Pollak, MB, FRCS, FACS
Associate Professor of Surgery
Chief, Division of Transplantation
University of Illinois at Chicago
Chief, Division of Transplantation
University of Illinois Hospitals and Clinics
Chicago, Illinois

Pedro A. Rivas, MD, MS
Research Associate
Department of Surgery
University of Illinois at Chicago
Chicago, Illinois

William D. Soper, MD
Assistant Professor of Surgery
Northwestern University Medical School
Attending Surgeon
Northwestern Memorial Hospital
Chicago, Illinois

Jonathan B. Towne, MD
Professor of Surgery
Medical College of Wisconsin
Chairman, Vascular Surgery
John L. Doyne Hospital
Milwaukee, Wisconsin

Mark Vajaranant, MD
Assistant Professor of Obstetrics and Gynecology
University of Illinois College of Medicine
University of Illinois Hospital and Clinics
Chicago, Illinois

Joseph M. Vitello, MD
Assistant Professor of Surgery
University of Illinois College of Medicine
Attending Surgeon
West Side Veterans Hospital
Chicago, Illinois

Preface

The first edition of Abdominal Pain was published 25 years ago under the senior editorship of Professor Lars-Erik Gelin of Gothenberg, Sweden. Although the first presentation was widely acclaimed, the premature death of Dr. Gelin in 1980 and the "pulls and tugs" of the expanding academic responsibilities of Drs. Condon and Nyhus prevented a revision until now. Dr. Joseph M. Vitello has joined us in this new effort.

The present monograph is based on an earlier Scandinavian work, Akut Abdomen, Kopenhamn: Bibliotheca Medica, 1960, produced by Dr. Gelin and on our own first English edition of 1969.

The emphasis on a detailed analysis of the information presented by a patient—symptoms of pain and other complaints and the signs noted on physical examination—is maintained in this edition. New to this edition, however, are chapters that describe specific disease entities that usually cause abdominal pain. We note areas of interest usually not highlighted in texts such as this, such as the role of laparoscopy, abdominal trauma, immunocompromise, and nonsurgical causes of abdominal pain.

This monograph does not replace the need for reading in depth on this subject in major textbooks of surgery. Rather we view our presentation as an additional guide for the rapid and accurate diagnosis of disorders that cause acute abdominal pain. When one has the correct diagnosis, the therapeutic approach usually is clear.

Professor Gelin and Dr. Nyhus studied with Professor Philip Sandblom in Lund, Sweden, in 1955. The current editors dedicate this edition to Lars-Erik Gelin, truly one of the great academic surgeons of the twentieth century.

We have many to thank for the development of this monograph. First, we thank our contributing authors, who stem from the Departments of Surgery of the University of Illinois College of Medicine at Chicago and the Medical College of Wisconsin in Milwaukee. Drs. Nyhus and Vitello thank Catherine Judge Allen and June Svec for organizing the manuscripts. Dr. Condon thanks Barbara Boye for being of major support. Finally, our friends at Appleton & Lange, Jane Licht and Ed Wickland, have been particularly understanding and helpful.

Lloyd M. Nyhus
Robert E. Condon
Joseph M. Vitello

CHAPTER 1

■

The Patient's Complaints and What They Mean

Joseph M. Vitello, MD
and Lloyd M. Nyhus, MD

The word *symptom* derives from the Greek and literally means "anything that has befallen one." Before the physician delves into the physical examination, the historical account and symptom complex of the problem should be procured and analyzed, not just for rote or documentation, but for guidance during the examination. The chronologic order in which the symptoms occur has distinct relevance and should be noted in detail. This seemingly trivial point is often lost in the enthusiasm to begin palpation of the abdomen. Since pain is often the chief complaint of patients presenting with abdominal disorders, it is dealt with in detail. Other symptoms, however, commonly accompany abdominal pain and these may or may not be integral components of the underlying pathologic conditions.

PAIN

Pain is a subjective experience, which the physician must be able to understand and interpret. The ability of the patient to reveal his or her symptoms is based on the individual's skills of communication and intelligence. Virtually all patients need direction and prompting during the procurement of the history to direct the course of the interview. The interviewer's ability to extract seemingly minute details of the history is only learned over time. The astute clinician knows from experience which important details and pain patterns help lead to the diagnosis. Since urgent intervention is often necessary when dealing with acute abdominal pain, experience and judgment must be developed and exercised so that the catastrophe of delay is averted.

The correct interpretation of acute abdominal pain becomes one of the most challenging demands placed upon the physician. Simplistically, determining the cause of a patient's abdominal pain may be likened to a jigsaw puzzle. Pieces of the puzzle are assembled, some fit together, others are incongruous. Ideally, enough "pieces" are arranged in an orderly fashion so that the remaining "puzzle" is easily solved, even with the absence of some parts.

Pain cannot be directly measured, as blood pressure is with a sphygmomanometer; what is intense pain for one patient may represent a mild discomfort to the stoic. Careful observation of the changes in the development, character, intensity, and localization of pain are essential. Optimally, the operating surgeon should be the one who examines the patient early and repeatedly. This not only improves rapport between patient and physician but affords the surgeon the opportunity to expand his or her skills in detecting abdominal pathologic conditions and correlating them with operative findings. These observations are best carried out without the use of analgesics, which tend to cloud the clinical picture. Reliable patients can usually accept this if they are told that it is in their best interest that analgesics be withheld until the diagnosis is secure. Because patients differ in their response to pain, occasionally an individual may benefit from a narcotic *prior* to the physical examination. This may convert an unreliable or difficult examination into a more achievable task. It is unlikely that a few milligrams of morphine will mask peritonitis, and the calming effect on the patient may create an environment more favorable for a dependable history and examination. The decision to administer an analgesic prior to examination should be made by the operating surgeon. Obviously, once the decision to operate has been made, there is no logical reason to withhold pain medications.

Origin of the Pain

Pain impulses originating in the abdominal cavity are transmitted via both the autonomic and the anterior and lateral spinothalamic tracts. Pain impulses conducted via the spinothalamic tracts are characterized easily and with good localization. This is the pain of *parietal* peritoneal irritation. The patient will commonly locate this pain at an exact spot with one or two fingers. This is achievable because the pain is transmitted by overlapping somatic nerves that innervate the peritoneum. Less often, localized pain is indicated with the whole hand, but in a limited, local, sweeping motion. This kind of pain is generally the result of an intra-abdominal inflammatory process that extends to or involves the parietal peritoneum. To correctly interpret the origin of localized pain, it is essential to think anatomically (Figs. 1 and 2). Pain impulses arising from intra-abdominal organs via the autonomic nervous system are due to ischemia, stretching or distention of a viscus, or peristaltic contraction of smooth muscle against a luminal obstruction. Such stimuli often give rise to poorly localized, diffuse pain in the center of the abdomen. This is commonly referred to as *visceral* peritoneal irritation. The patient often delineates this pain by passing the opened hand in a circular fashion over

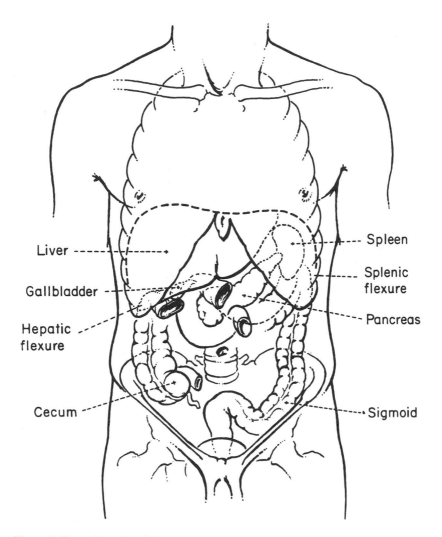

Liver

Gallbladder

Hepatic
flexure

Cecum

Spleen

Splenic
flexure

Pancreas

Sigmoid

Figure 1. Normal location of the major viscera in relation to anterior anatomic landmarks.

the entire abdomen or a large part of it. Visceral pain may be felt in the epigastric, umbilical, or pubic regions. The patient is usually unable to further localize the pain or be more descriptive about it. Interestingly, the intestine can be cut, burned, or crushed without the patient experiencing the sensation of pain.

The segmental anatomic relationships between the autonomic and the spinothalamic nerves often give rise to referral of visceral pain. Localized

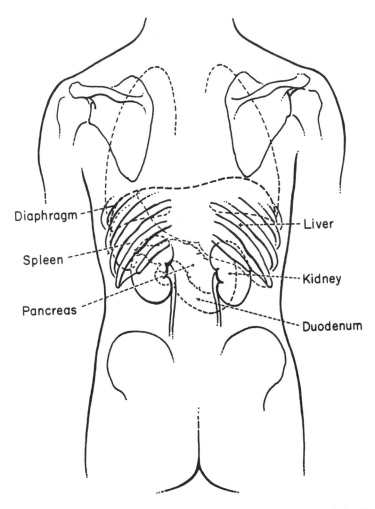

Figure 2. Normal location of certain viscera in relation to posterior anatomic landmarks.

pain does not always exist precisely where the problem lies, since pain may be referred to a point outside the abdomen. For example, perforating ulcer, pleurisy, hemoperitoneum, or subphrenic abscess may irritate the diaphragm. The pain impulses are carried via the phrenic nerve to the fourth cervical segment. The pain is then perceived in (referred to) the sensory area also supplied by C4, the top of the shoulder or lateral aspect of the neck. Often this information is of diagnostic value. The pathways of such pain referrals are not always well defined, but the clinical pattern is reliable enough to make it

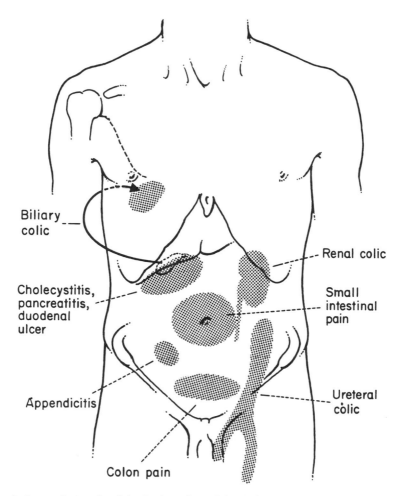

Figure 3. Areas where pain originating in various abdominal structures is perceived or referred.

useful. Thus, pain radiating toward a certain area may suggest a specific diagnosis (Figs. 3 and 4), for example:

Left shoulder region	pancreatitis, left pleural or cardiac disease, splenic injury, perforated ulcer
Right shoulder region	perforated ulcer, right-sided pleurisy, subphrenic abscess, splenic injury
Right subscapular region	biliary disease

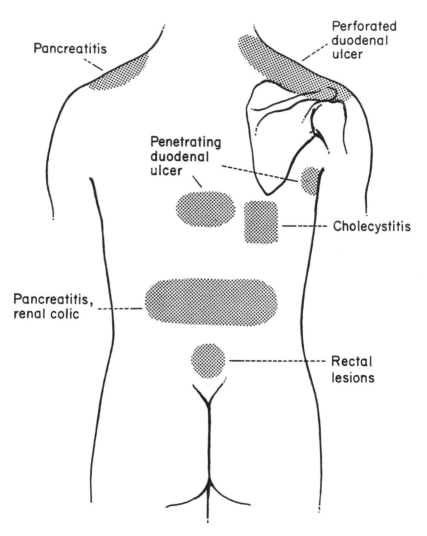

Figure 4. Posterior areas where abdominal pain is perceived or referred.

Inguinal and genital area	urogenital disease, appendicitis, inguinal hernia
Sacrum	diseases of the genitalia or rectum

Analysis of Pain

In the majority of patients with acute abdominal pain, a careful analysis of the problem is sufficient for a reliable diagnosis. In some circumstances, an exact diagnosis is irrelevant, since the patient presents with clear indications for operation. With many diseases, the pain follows certain patterns that are almost pathognomonic. Pain should be analyzed with regard to the following nine factors: (1) onset, (2) progression, (3) migration, (4) character, (5) intensity, (6) localization and radiation, (7) duration, (8) exacerbating conditions, and finally, (9) alleviating conditions. While this analysis seems laborious, the physician is rewarded by often reaching the diagnosis without needing expensive radiologic tests or excessive laboratory investigation.

Onset. Acute pain may be produced by the new onset of a disease, such as appendicitis, or by the sudden exacerbation of a chronic problem, as in perforation of a preexisting duodenal ulcer or gangrenous cholecystitis resulting from known biliary calculi. Many abdominal pain syndromes are heralded by prodromal symptoms such as dyspepsia before perforation of an ulcer or syncope associated with rupture of an ectopic pregnancy or aortic aneurysm. In other patients, acute pain occurs in an isolated fashion, without warning and in the absence of previous symptoms.

The minute and hour of the onset of acute pain should be noted and considered in relation to the time of examination and commencement of treatment. The time interval between pain onset and examination is important in evaluating the symptoms and development of the disease (Table 1). The pain of an acutely perforated ulcer is of such an intense nature that the average person seeks medical attention within minutes. A patient with acute sigmoid diverticulitis may wait many hours or even a few days before realizing the situation is not improving. The relationship of the onset of the pain to meals may have importance, as with cholecystitis or ulcer disease. The time of day at which the pain occurs should be ascertained, since it may have diagnostic connotations, as with the nocturnal pain of duodenal ulcer.

TABLE 1. DIAGNOSTIC PATTERNS OF THE ONSET OF PAIN

Features	Sudden	Gradual	Slow
Begins	Within seconds to minutes	Within minutes to hours, days	Insidiously (days to weeks)
Patient's recollection of onset	Exact; within minutes	Close; within an hour	Vague (hours to days)
Maximum intensity	At onset	After a short interval (minutes to hours)	After a long interval (hours to days)
Typical description by patient relates onset to	A precise event	Activity during onset	Length of time pain has been present

Sudden Onset (Seconds to Minutes). This type of pain occurs immediately, reaching maximum intensity at once. Patients usually indicate the sudden onset by describing its occurrence with whatever they were doing at the time. Patients tend to be quite descriptive and precise about the onset of the pain, eg: "I was at the office and had just finished some paper work, got up from my desk, and that's when the pain hit me." Or the patient may have noted the exact minute at which the pain originated. Sudden onset of pain is typical of ulcer perforation, ruptured aortic aneurysm, or testicular or ovarian torsion (Fig. 5, Table 2).

Gradual Onset (Minutes to Hours to a Few Days). This pain commences within a few minutes and increases in severity during the next several hours or days. Maximal pain is reached not at onset but after a short interval. A typical description might be: "I was at the office and began to have abdominal

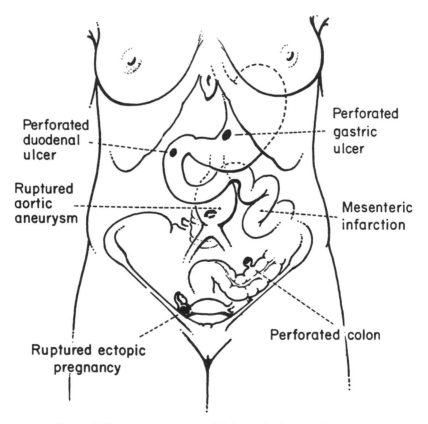

Figure 5. The common causes of abdominal pain of sudden onset.

TABLE 2. CAUSES OF PAIN OF ACUTE ONSET

Perforated duodenal or gastric ulcer
Intra-abdominal rupture of an abscess or hematoma
Ruptured esophagus
Ruptured ectopic pregnancy
Spontaneous pneumothorax
Ruptured aortic abdominal aneurysm
Aortic dissection
Rectus sheath hematoma
Ruptured intervertebral disk
Testicular or ovarian torsion
RARELY:
Acute appendicitis
Acute cholecystitis
Ureteral stone

pain sometime in the morning. I continued to work, but by the afternoon it became so severe I went to the emergency room." Gradual onset is a common pain pattern that occurs with a variety of acute abdominal diseases such as acute cholecystitis, appendicitis, pancreatitis, nonperforated diverticulitis, and uncomplicated small-intestinal obstruction (Fig. 6, Table 3). Acute mesenteric thrombosis or embolus tends to produce a pain pattern that fits into this category more frequently than in the acute-onset one.

Slowly Developing Onset (Days to Weeks). This designation applies to pain that becomes severe only after many hours or even days have passed. The patient is usually vague as to the actual onset of the pain. Slowly developing pain may be described as: "The pain began a couple of days ago; yesterday I stayed home from work hoping it would improve, but it hasn't." This pattern is more common with visceral neoplasms, chronic inflammatory conditions, and malignant colonic obstruction. It is occasionally seen with appendicitis, especially when the initial presentation was misdiagnosed.

Onset After Trauma. Many patients relate the onset of pain to a recent episode of blunt trauma. It is important to learn the time of onset of the pain as well as when the injury occurred. If the timing coincides, rupture of a solid or hollow organ must be considered. Many times the association of pain onset with a minor episode of trauma is only coincidental and thus tends to obscure the true underlying pathologic condition. An example is the patient who complains of back pain after lifting a heavy object and also notes weight loss and early satiety; these are all symptoms of occult pancreatic cancer, not a lower-back injury.

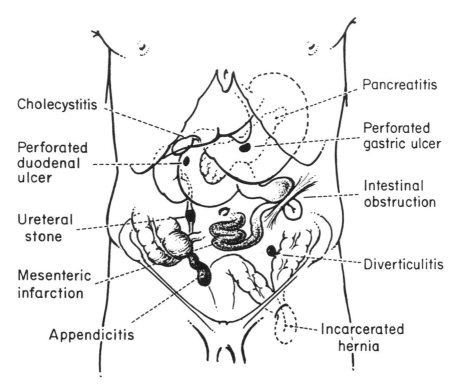

Figure 6. The common causes of abdominal pain of gradual onset.

TABLE 3. CAUSES OF ABDOMINAL PAIN OF GRADUAL ONSET

Acute urinary retention	Mesenteric lymphadenitis
Appendicitis	Pancreatitis
Cholecystitis	Perforated tumor (usually of
Cystitis or pyelonephritis	the colon or stomach)
Duodenal ulcer	Prostatic vesiculitis
Ectopic pregnancy before rupture	Salpingo-oophoritis (PID)
Gastric dilatation	Sigmoid diverticulitis
Gastric ulcer	Small-intestinal tumor or infarct
Gastritis	Strangulated hernia
Intra-abdominal abscess	Terminal ileitis (regional
Low, mechanical small-intestinal	enteritis; Crohn's disease)
obstruction	Threatening abortion
Meckel's diverticulitis	Ulcerative colitis
Mesenteric cyst	Ureteral stone colic

Progression. Questions of vital interest to the physician should include: Has the pain subsided or increased? Have there been periods of time when the patient is totally pain free? Has the pain changed in character? A perforated ulcer may spontaneously become plugged with omentum and with time the pain, tenderness, and muscular spasms disappear. The patient may feel improved and have minimal physical findings. Hours later, if the omentum recedes, the pain will recur. With a mechanical intestinal obstruction, if the blockage is partially relieved, the pain will diminish or vanish, only to return later if worsening obstruction occurs. Alternatively, the adhesive small-intestinal obstruction that began as intense crampy pain may now progress to moderately severe, constant pain as blood supply to the intestine is compromised and strangulation occurs. Sometimes the prodrome of appendicitis is a diffuse, rather severe, intermittent pain similar to that of intestinal obstruction. These pains subside and are followed by a gradually increasing, localized, dull ache in the right lower abdomen.

It is erroneous to assume that the subsidence of severe symptoms indicates the disease is regressing. The pain of appendicitis is commonly thought to improve temporarily as the organ perforates, relieving the pressure of the obstructing fecalith. With nasogastric tube decompression and intravenous hydration, the patient with an adhesive small-intestinal obstruction may feel improved, but persistent obstipation suggests the need for operation.

Migration. Pain migration implies that the original location of the perceived discomfort moves to a different site during the early-to-mid course of the illness. This phenomenon occurs most often and typically with appendicitis. In this condition, the pain commences in the mid abdomen and after some time moves to the right lower quadrant and localizes over McBurney's point. Migration of pain can also occur with perforated ulcer, the pain initially being epigastric, later right lower quadrant or pelvic in location. In sigmoid diverticulitis, pain commences around the umbilicus and settles in the left lower quadrant. Migration of pain may be confused with radiation of pain, which is also common with abdominal disease. The distinction is that with migration, the discomfort starts in one location, seemingly resolves, and then a new, more intense pain occurs in a contiguous location. Radiation implies that the moderately severe initial discomfort is continuous and associated with a secondary, possibly noncontiguous location of equal or lesser pain. The classic example of pain radiation is the left shoulder pain noted with diaphragmatic irritation.

Character. The character of pain gives the best clue to understanding the pathophysiologic aspects of an acute abdomen. Many adjectives are employed to aid in the description and documentation of pain. Burning, cramping, stabbing, gnawing, pricking, boring, and aching are all terms that are used to describe the quality of pain. Simplistically if not practically, pain is

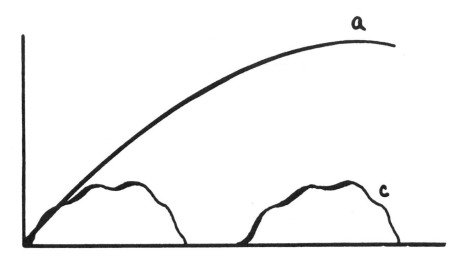

Figure 7. Aching (toothache) pain steadily rises to a maximum intensity (a). This pattern of aching pain is seen in the inflammation of solid viscera and with late ischemic changes in obstructed hollow viscera. Cramps (c) are short episodes of mild pain and are typical of early inflammation of a hollow viscus.

most easily characterized as either constant or intermittent (colicky) and, secondly, as superficial or deep.

Crampy or Colicky Pain. Crampy or colicky pain is a short-term, poorly localized episode of distress (Fig. 7, Table 4). Mild cramps are usually of no surgical significance and are noted by most people at some time in their life. More severe cramps may indicate irritation, obstruction, or mild inflammation of viscera. Cramps produced by intra-abdominal disease of a serious nature will often change character to a constant, severe ache.

Intermittent Colicky Pain. The pain increases in severity in short waves to a maximum and then abruptly ceases, to be followed by an entirely pain-free interval of short or long duration. The cycle then repeats itself (Fig. 8). This type of pain is commonly caused by a mechanical intestinal obstruction. The duration of the pain-free interval often indicates the anatomic site of the obstruction. The more proximal the obstruction, the shorter the pain-free interval. The more distal the obstruction, the longer the pain-free interval.

Continuous Colicky Pain. This type of pain is similar to intermittent colic, but pain-free intervals are lacking. The intensity of pain can be depicted as a toothed sine curve that never returns to the base line (Fig. 9). This type of pain

TABLE 4. DIFFERENTIAL DIAGNOSIS OF COLICKY PAIN

Involved Organ	Free Interval?	Common Cause	Other Major Symptoms or Signs	Helpful Diagnostic Examinations	Initial Treatment
Stomach	None	Pyloric obstruction	Vomiting	UGI Series	NG suction; operation
	None	Gastritis	Vomiting, bleeding, pain	Endoscopy	Medical management
Small Intestine	1–5 min or less	Mechanical obstruction	Vomiting	Radiographs: flat and upright	NG suction; operation
	1–5 min	Enteritis; paralytic ileus	Diarrhea; distention	Radiographs: flat and upright	NG suction, hydration
Large Intestine	5–20 min	Mechanical obstruction	Distention	Radiographs: flat and upright LGI	Operation
	3–5 min	Colitis	Diarrhea	Endoscopy	Hydration, nutritional support
Appendix	None	Inflammation	Pain migration	Ultrasound LGI	Operation
Bile ducts	None (usually)	Stone	Vomiting	Cholangiogram ERCP	Operation, sphincterotomy
		Stricture	Jaundice	Cholangiogram	Operation, stent
Pancreas	None	Stone (CBD)	Jaundice	Amylase (high)	Operation, ERCP, stent
	Short or absent	Inflammation; necrosis	Abdominal pain Hypovolemia	Computed tomography	Hydration, bowel rest, nutritional support
Kidneys and ureters	Variable	Stone	Hematuria	IVP	Analgesics
Testis	None	Torsion	Tender scrotal mass	Scrotal Doppler	Operation
Uterus and tubes	2–5 min	Abortion	Hemorrhage	Vaginal: open cervix	Curettage
	1–5 min or absent	Dysmenorrhea	—	Laparoscopy	Analgesics

CBD, common bile duct; ERCP, endoscopic retrograde cholangiopancreatography; IVP, intravenous pyelography; LGI, lower gastrointestinal study; NG, nasogastric; UGI, upper gastrointestinal.

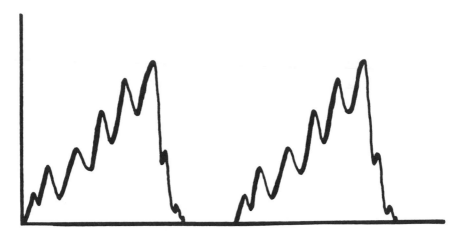

Figure 8. Intermittent colicky pain increases in waves to a maximum and then rapidly relents. There is no or very minimal discomfort until the next cycle begins. This pain pattern is very common early in obstruction of a hollow viscus.

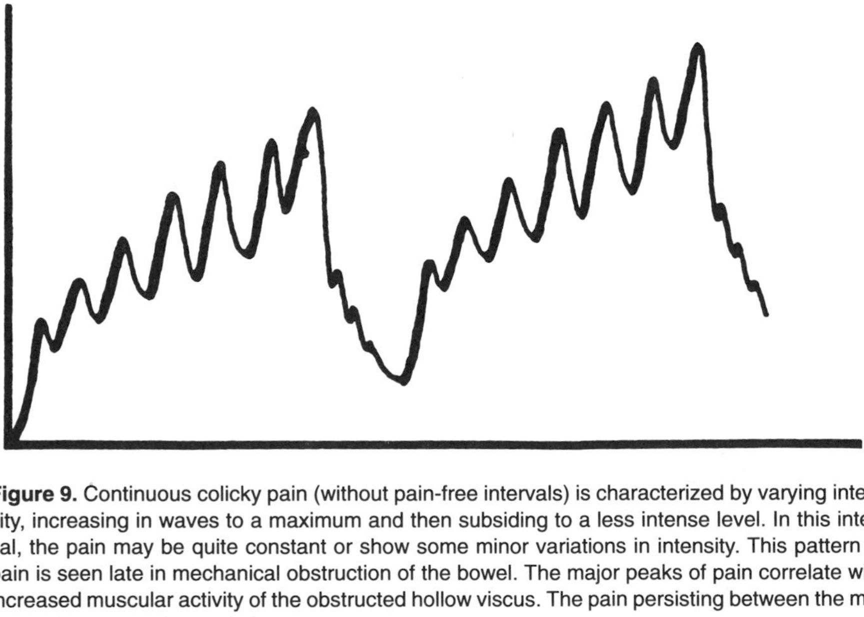

Figure 9. Continuous colicky pain (without pain-free intervals) is characterized by varying intensity, increasing in waves to a maximum and then subsiding to a less intense level. In this interval, the pain may be quite constant or show some minor variations in intensity. This pattern of pain is seen late in mechanical obstruction of the bowel. The major peaks of pain correlate with increased muscular activity of the obstructed hollow viscus. The pain persisting between the major peaks is related to early ischemia.

occurs most commonly with biliary or renal stones, high small-intestinal obstruction, and intestinal strangulation.

Constant Ache. Distress of this type is usually compared to a toothache. It can be pictured as a curve steadily rising in intensity (Fig. 7A). Constant, aching pain usually is caused by a marked swelling or overdistention of a hollow viscus or by impending or actual ischemia and gangrene. The intensity of the pain is related to the degree of swelling or ischemia but ultimately becomes quite severe. This is typically the characteristic pain noted in acute pancreatitis or localized, suppurative appendicitis.

Anxiety and Pain. Anxiety reactions related to severe pain vary from patient to patient. Some degree of anxiety will be found in individuals predisposed to this sort of reaction, no matter what kind or degree of pain they suffer. Recognition of the anxiety-prone patient is an important factor in correctly interpreting symptoms. Anxiety typically accompanies the pain of acute myocardial infarction (MI) and acute pancreatitis, even in stoic patients. With MI, the patient will often want to sit up. The patient with pancreatitis will often be retching and curled up in a fetal position. Perforated ulcer and peritonitis are associated with less anxiety, since the patient tends to lie quite still to avoid the exacerbation of pain through movement. Patients with renal colic suffer very severe pains and consequently look very anxious. These patients are diaphoretic, writhing, vomiting, and miserable. It is the severely anxious individual, from whom the history or physical examination is difficult to obtain, who occasionally benefits from a narcotic prior to the examination.

The Relation of Pain to Respiration. If pain increases with deep inspiration, it may indicate a disease condition near the diaphragm. This type of abdominal pain can be caused by pleuritis, basilar pneumonia, pulmonary embolus, or subphrenic irritation from cholecystitis or a perforated ulcer.

Depth of Pain. Oftentimes the patient can distinguish between a deep-seated pain or a sensation that the pain is superficial. Pain felt to be "deep" more commonly arises from a visceral organ without associated parietal peritoneal irritation. The pain of pancreatic neoplasm fits into this category well. More superficial pain is noted with problems that are anatomically close to the anterior abdominal wall. Examples include an anteriorly located appendicitis, abdominal wall hernias, rectus sheath hematoma, and nerve entrapment syndromes. Although this categorization may be of limited help, it is one that is often overlooked; fortunately it is easily reproducable from one examiner to the next.

Intensity. Since pain is a subjective experience, the intensity cannot be measured and depends, in part, on the individual's perception and response. The patient is often asked to liken his or her pain to a common discernable event to which most people can relate: the pain of a toothache, childbirth, gas cramps, etc. The patient's behavior and visual cues during pain usually clarify its intensity better than the patient's verbal description. Individuals who appear to be relaxed and comfortably watching television when the examiner approaches, only to begin moaning with pain, should be suspected of malingering. It should be noted whether the patient's facial expression mirrors the subjective report of pain. The history should include information as to whether the patient has continued daily work despite the pain. Other matters of question include: does the patient have to lie down because of the pain? Did the pain prevent sleep or awaken the patient? Does the patient cry out or groan because of the severity of the pain? Does the patient lie still or writhe about? Writhing about is more characteristic of pain arising in a hollow viscus, or from ischemia, whereas lying still is more characteristic of peritonitis. Other vital signs will often be aberrant during severe abdominal pain, such as shortness of breath and elevation of pulse, temperature, and blood pressure. The intensity of pain is dependent on the type and degree of foreign substance that is initiating the pain or irritating the intraperitoneal contents. Caustic substances such as hydrochloric acid (HCL) even in small amounts, spilled into the abdominal cavity after an ulcer perforates, causes severe, instantaneous abdominal pain. Limited volumes of blood or bile may cause much less severe pain initially. The volume of irritant is also of importance, since a large volume of HCL will lead to the diffuse, boardlike rigidity typically noted with a perforated ulcer. A small inoculum of bacteria from a fishbone perforation of the small intestine may initially cause trivial pain. Once bacterial proliferation occurs, an inflammatory response ensues, and more severe pain is experienced.

At the simplest, it may be recorded whether the patient perceives the pain as mild, moderate, or severe. Individual variation will occur. Certain disease entities have varying intensities of pain, even during the normal course of the illness. Some physicians ask the patient to grade the severity of pain on a scale of 1 to 10. However, this scale probably does not have any practical significance. In general, mild pain often is insignificant. But the progression of mild pain to moderate or severe pain is an important differential. However, most patients do not seek medical attention or enjoy waiting in an emergency room in the middle of the night for the evaluation of a mild pain. Typically, the patient who perceives that his pain is unusual will seek evaluation. Early on, physical findings may be minimal, yet the patient is truly ill. This is typical for appendicitis. In contradistinction, the pain of a perforated ulcer or ureteral colic is so severe as to humble even the most stoic individual. To illustrate the scale of progression, the pain of early appendicitis is mild, McBurney's point tenderness and parietal peritoneal irritation bring on moderate tenderness, and finally perforation and peritonitis complete the spectrum and are perceived as severe pain in most patients.

Localization and Radiation. Localized pain is a sign of inflammation of the parietal peritoneum. With cholecystitis, pain often occurs below the right rib margin; with pyelonephritis, over the involved kidney; with appendicitis, in the right iliac fossa; and so forth.

Radiating pain is of particular diagnostic value (Figs. 3 and 4). With biliary colic, there is often radiation of pain around the side and to the right subscapular region; with renal colic, pain radiates down toward the groin and urethra; and with cardiac pain, radiation is toward the left shoulder. Radiation of pain often occurs as a result of irritation of a segmental nerve. This occurs with herpes zoster when a single nerve distribution is involved. A herniated intervertebral disk may lead to an anatomically distinct lancinating pain as a single spinal nerve root is compressed. Another mechanism explaining the radiation of pain has to do with an organ's embryologic origin. Phrenic pain is an important type of referred pain that fits into this category. With irritation of the diaphragm, which embryologically is innervated by spinal nerves derived from C4, pain may be perceived at the top of the shoulder and base of the neck. This may occur with such conditions as cholecystitis, perforating ulcer, a subphrenic abscess, injured spleen, and sometimes with pelvic inflammatory disease. Other times, pain radiation occurs because of anatomic proximity to other organs. Sometimes the mechanism of pain radiation is unclear.

Duration. Fleeting pains that come and go tend to be inconsequential, whereas pain occurring over the course of several hours or days tends to be more pathologic and related to true disease. Pain of weeks' or months' duration, especially with associated weight loss or lassitude, is commonly associated with an underlying malignant neoplasm. Pain of months' or years' duration, without associated symptoms, leads to skepticism on the part of the examiner but on occasion has anatomic basis.

Exacerbation or Alleviation

The Patient's Position. A deep breath may worsen any pain, if diaphragmatic irritation exists. Therefore, observation of the patient during a deep inspiration may be of value. Alternatively, the dyspneic patient may be short of breath not because of pulmonary disease but rather because of a subdiaphragmatic process. Patients with peritonitis, regardless of the underlying mechanism, tend to lie motionless, since movement will exacerbate their pain. The car ride to the hospital or a trip to the radiology department can be distinctly uncomfortable when a bump is encountered. Coughing, laughing, walking, or even sitting up may be difficult. This is in contradistinction to the patient with mesenteric ischemia who writhes and rolls about in bed with excruciating pain, unable to become comfortable regardless of position. Patients with pancreatitis are commonly curled up in a fetal position to alleviate the pressure of the retroperitoneal organ on surrounding structures. Psoas irritation, as in retrocecal appendicitis, will cause the patient to lie supine with the right leg flexed at the hip and knee. Patients with renal colic will often look miserable, be sitting up in bed, hunched over an emesis basin because of their protracted vomiting and wretching. Seemingly no position can alleviate their pain.

Relationship to Meals. It often helps to know whether the ingestion of food initiates or worsen the pain (cholecystitis and pancreatitis), or improves and eliminates the pain (ulcer), or if the patient is nauseated by food and anorectic (appendicitis).

Effect of Medications. Often the patient has attempted to medicate him- or herself, with varying degrees of success or failure. Aspirin or related compounds may worsen the pain of ulcers or gastritis and has no effect on peritonitis. A tablet or elixir of antacid may alleviate the pain of ulcers yet be ineffectual in cholecystitis. Sublingual nitroglycerin may relieve not only the pain of ischemic heart disease but also cholelithiasis or reflux esophagitis.

Age of the Patient

Since the prevalence of certain pathologic entities is more common at specific ages of life, this factor should be taken into account. Intussusception is more common under the age of two, appendicitis occurs in adolescents and young adults, and colonic obstruction is seen more in the older population. While exceptions abound, the age of the patient is another piece of the puzzle that may aid in detecting the cause of the abdominal pain.

Location of Pain

Pain is usually either diffuse or localized, which as mentioned previously has prognostic implications as to its source. Certain viscera provide reasonably good localization of pain, whereas others afford little information. If pain is confined to a specific region, anatomic considerations are the logical starting point. Too often, in the differential diagnosis of a pain, the inexperienced physician fails to consider the anatomic structures directly beneath or in proximity to the area of tenderness. Next, the referral of pain from another area should be considered. This mental exercise should be constantly practiced as each new patient presents with an episode of abdominal pain. There are three major areas in the abdomen where pain of visceral origin occurs: the epigastrium, the region around the umbilicus, and the suprapubic and pelvic region.

Pain in the Upper or Middle Abdomen. Pain in the epigastrium usually arises from disease processes in the heart, lungs, pleurae, liver, bile ducts, pancreas, stomach, duodenum, or spleen. It may, however, arise from the small intestine, appendix, or colon (Figs. 10 and 11, Table 5). The most common causes of

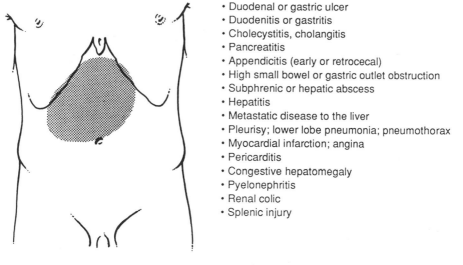

- Duodenal or gastric ulcer
- Duodenitis or gastritis
- Cholecystitis, cholangitis
- Pancreatitis
- Appendicitis (early or retrocecal)
- High small bowel or gastric outlet obstruction
- Subphrenic or hepatic abscess
- Hepatitis
- Metastatic disease to the liver
- Pleurisy; lower lobe pneumonia; pneumothorax
- Myocardial infarction; angina
- Pericarditis
- Congestive hepatomegaly
- Pyelonephritis
- Renal colic
- Splenic injury

Figure 10. The common causes of upper abdominal pain.

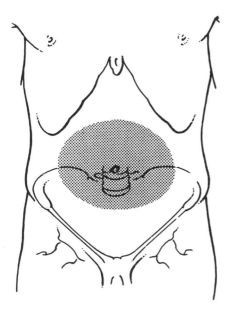

- Appendicitis (early)
- Small intestinal obstruction or gangrene
- Pancreatitis
- Gastroenteritis
- Mesenteric embolus/thrombosis
- Umbilical hernia
- Aortic abdominal aneurysm
- Aortic dissection
- Sigmoid diverticulitis (early)
- Mesenteric adenitis

Figure 11. The common causes of periumbilical or midabdominal pain.

TABLE 5. DIFFERENTIAL DIAGNOSIS OF PAIN IN THE UPPER OR MIDABDOMEN

Involved Organ	Common Cause	Major Symptoms and Signs	Helpful Examinations	Initial Treatment
Stomach and duodenum	Perforation	Muscular guarding, rigid abdomen	Abdominal radiographs (free air in 80%)	Hydration, operation
	Penetrating ulcer	Decreased pain with food or antacid	Endoscopy, UGI series	Medication, analgesics
Bile ducts	Cholelithiasis	Vomiting, RUQ pain	Ultrasound	Hydration, elective operation
	Cholecystitis	Fever, palpable gallbladder, (+) Murphy's sign	Ultrasound, HIDA scan	Operation
	Cholangitis	Fever, jaundice, RUQ pain	—	Antibiotics, operation
Pancreas	Inflammation, necrosis	Vomiting, epigastric pain, shock	Serum amylase, CT scan	Hydration
Appendix	Inflammation	Pain migration, McBurney's point tenderness	Ultrasound, LGI examination	Operation
Lungs	Pneumonia	Fever, dyspnea	Chest radiograph	Antibiotics
	Pleurisy	Dyspnea, chest pain	Chest radiograph	Analgesics
	Pneumothorax	Dyspnea	Chest radiograph	Chest tube
Heart	Infarction	Anxiety, dyspnea, radiating chest pain	ECG, cardiac enzymes	Cardiology consultation
	Angina	Anxiety, dyspnea, radiating chest pain	ECG, cardiac enzymes	Nitroglycerin, cardiology consultation
	Congestive failure	Edema, hepatomegaly, JVD	Chest radiograph	Diuretics, inotropes, cardiology consultation

CT, computerized tomography; ECG, electrocardiogram; HIDA, hepatobiliary scan; JVD, jugular vein distention; LGI, lower gastrointestinal; RUQ, right upper quadrant; UGI, upper gastrointestinal.

epigastric pain are cholecystitis, penetrating or perforated duodenal or gastric ulcer, and appendicitis. If the cause is gastric or duodenal, pain is felt in the midepigastrium or subxiphoid region, and there is often a history of chronic dyspepsia prior to the attack of acute pain. Muscular guarding and tenderness in the epigastrium are virtually always found with perforation. Radiographs show free air in approximately 80% of instances.

A penetrating ulcer induces pain in the epigastrium, which often radiates to the back between the scapulae and worsens with fasting or at night. The pain usually diminishes if the patient drinks a glass of milk or eats some food, producing neutralization of the acid. Posterior penetration of the ulcer does not lead to muscular guarding, but tenderness is often noted on deep palpation of the epigastric region.

An acute duodenal ulcer causes pain in the epigastrium. Vomiting may occur as a result of pylorospasm or gastric outlet obstruction. The pain may be intense but seldom leads to muscular guarding unless perforation has occurred.

Acute gastric dilatation can occur spontaneously and without anatomic obstruction to the emptying of the stomach. Persistent pain, which may radiate to the left shoulder, hiccups, and a distended upper abdomen with a succussion splash dominate the clinical signs and symptoms. Hypotension may rarely be present.

If the epigastric pain originates in the biliary tract, the pain generally radiates under the right costal arch toward the subscapular region. If choledocholithiasis exists, the pain is constant, with intermittent peaks. Rarely is the pain so intense that the patient is writhing. Vomiting is not uncommon but usually is not protracted. The abdomen may be soft, although some degree of guarding and tenderness is usual. Fever above 101°F is uncommon with an uncomplicated common bile duct stone. Jaundice varies, depending on the degree of obstruction and the period of time that has elapsed since the stone migrated into the common duct. Gradual dilatation of the biliary tree, as may occur with carcinoma of the head of the pancreas, may be painless.

With acute cholecystitis, ie, cystic duct obstruction, pain is more constant, not colicky as commonly described, and localized under the right costal margin. The intensity of pain reflects the degree of circulatory disturbance in the gallbladder wall. Fever is generally low grade (<100°F) and occurs after 12 to 24 hours. Localized tenderness occurs in the right upper quadrant and the gallbladder may be palpable. In some patients, however, the inflamed gallbladder is covered by ribs or omentum and not palpable, but an inspiratory arrest occurs when the patient is asked to take a deep breath and the examiner simultaneously palpates the right upper quadrant (Murphy's sign).

With acute parenchymal liver disease, like hepatitis from any cause, pain is more diffuse in the entire upper abdomen and is accompanied by anorexia. The aversion to food may be so marked that the mere thought of it leads to nausea. The intensity of pain is quite variable but rarely classified as severe.

The appearance of obvious jaundice usually occurs a few days after the first onset of pain. The liver is enlarged and tender and its rounded edge is easily felt in the soft and otherwise normal abdomen.

With pancreatitis, pain, like the overall disease picture, can be of varying character. While acute hemorrhagic or necrotizing pancreatitis usually presents with striking signs and symptoms, milder forms of pancreatitis more closely resemble biliary colic, angina pectoris, or gastroenteritis. Pancreatitis is manifested by colicky or constant pain in the epigastrium, radiating toward the left or right side. Typically the pain bores through to the back as though an arrow had pierced the patient's abdomen.

Recurring pancreatitis may also exist without simultaneous biliary disease. Often there is a history of alcohol abuse. Generally, this form of pancreatitis is characterized by moderately intense, constant or colicky pain, localizing to the epigastrium and radiating to the left upper quadrant and possibly the left shoulder and straight through to the back. A rise in the serum amylase is usually noted during the acute attack; however, a burned-out gland may not demonstrate biochemical aberrations. Calcifications noted within the pancreatic duct on plain film of the abdomen is a late finding in patients who have had multiple, recurrent attacks. Steatorrhea and glucose intolerance may be noted as a manifestation of pancreatic exocrine and endocrine insufficiency.

Appendicitis may start with pain localized exclusively in the upper portion of the abdomen. Later, the pain migrates and localizes below or around the umbilicus and ultimately in the right lower quadrant.

Colitis or colon obstruction can give rise to epigastric pain. This occurs most commonly when there is ischemia of the transverse colon with the threat of penetration or perforation.

With palpable splenomegaly there may be localized pain in the left upper quadrant and possible radiation to the left shoulder and neck. If a splenic infarct occurs, as in sickle cell patients, the pain becomes intense and severe, often with an associated fever and pleural effusion.

With high small-intestinal obstruction, pain localizes in the upper portion of the abdomen. Vomiting is usually quite prominent and the intensity of the colic frequent and severe.

When the cause of epigastric pain is pulmonary in origin, the pain is synchronized with respiratory efforts and combined with dyspnea. Pneumonia is usually accompanied by high fever and rales or dullness in the lungs. Chest roentgenography should confirm this diagnosis. Pleurisy may be present with or without fever. Pleuritic pain radiates toward the throat and shoulder and is exacerbated by deep breathing. Pain of a pleuritic nature may also be found with subphrenic irritation following ulcer perforation, cholecystitis, or pancreatitis. The diagnosis of pneumothorax is made by noting increased resonance on the side of the chest with diminished or absent breath sounds. Chest radiographs are confirmatory. A thorough physical examination of the chest with a quality radiograph should aid in establishing virtually all causes of abdominal pain originating from pulmonary pathologic phenomena.

If the cause of epigastric pain is cardiac in origin, the pain is usually associated with anxiety and sometimes dyspnea. Biliary colic and pancreatitis are often misinterpreted as angina pectoris and vice versa. Angina pectoris most often causes pain radiating toward the left arm and shoulder region or jaw. However, this is sufficiently variable that pain in and around the heart must be objectively excluded as cardiac in origin. Results of physical examination of the abdomen should be normal.

Acute myocardial infarction can give rise to conditions that resemble a perforated ulcer, cholecystitis, or pancreatitis. With peritonitis, the entire upper abdomen is tender, and pain is markedly increased by palpation. With myocardial infarction, the abdomen is not tender and pain is not exacerbated by abdominal palpation.

Cardiac failure may cause mild to moderate upper abdominal pain as a result of congestion of the liver and other viscera. Heart failure is almost always accompanied by dyspnea. Enlargement of the heart on chest radiograph, enlargement of the liver on abdominal palpation, and peripheral edema may all be present.

Pain in the Lower Abdomen. Pain below the umbilicus can arise from a variety of structures (Fig. 12, Table 6). It may also be caused by an exudate drain-

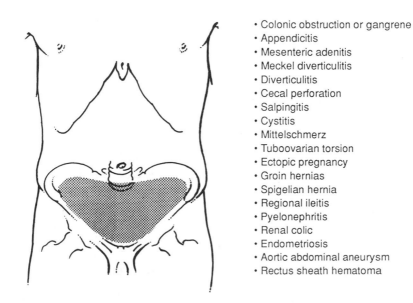

- Colonic obstruction or gangrene
- Appendicitis
- Mesenteric adenitis
- Meckel diverticulitis
- Diverticulitis
- Cecal perforation
- Salpingitis
- Cystitis
- Mittelschmerz
- Tuboovarian torsion
- Ectopic pregnancy
- Groin hernias
- Spigelian hernia
- Regional ileitis
- Pyelonephritis
- Renal colic
- Endometriosis
- Aortic abdominal aneurysm
- Rectus sheath hematoma

Figure 12. The common causes of pain in the lower abdomen and suprapubic region.

TABLE 6. DIFFERENTIAL DIAGNOSIS OF PAIN IN THE LOWER ABDOMEN*

Involved Organ	Common Cause	Other Major Symptoms and Signs	Helpful Examinations	Initial Treatment
Appendix	Inflammation	Epigastric or periumbilical pain at onset	Ultrasound LGI	Operation
Small Intestine	Obstruction (mechanical)	Vomiting, crampy pain, distention	Radiography	NG suction; operation
	Enteritis	Diarrhea	Endoscopy	NPO, hydration
	Ileus (paralytic)	Vomiting, distention	Radiography	NG suction, hydration
	Meckel's diverticulitis	Abdominal pain		Operation
	Lymphadenitis			—
	Obstructed or strangulated hernia	vomiting, palpation of tender hernial sac	—	Operation
Colon	Obstruction	Change in bowel habits	Radiography, LGI	Operation
	Diverticulitis	Fever, abdominal pain	Computed tomography	Antibiotics
	Colitis	Diarrhea	Endoscopy	Fast
Kidneys and Ureters	Pyelitis	Fever	Urinalysis; IVP	Antibiotics
	Stone	Hematuria	Urinalysis; IVP	Spasmolytics; analgesics
Bladder	Retention	Palpable bladder		Catheterization
	Cystitis	Urgent urination	Urinalysis	Antibiotics
Uterus and tubes	Ectopic pregnancy	Fainting	Vag.: soft mass	Operation
	Salpingitis	Fever	Vag.: tender mass	Antibiotics
	Abortion	Hemorrhage	Vag.: open cervix	Curettage
Ovaries	Twisted cyst	Shock	Vag.: firm, tender mass	Operation
	Follicular rupture	Fainting	Laparoscopy	Observation

*Always Perform *Rectal* and *Vaginal* Examination
IVP, intravenous pyelography; LGI, lower gastrointestinal; NG, nasogastric; NPO, nothing by mouth; vag, vagina.

ing from a disease process originating in the upper abdomen. Appendicitis typically begins with a dull central or periumbilical pain accompanied or preceded by anorexia. The pain then shifts, becoming localized in the right lower quadrant and associated with nausea, vomiting, and low-grade fever.

Incarcerated or strangulated hernia produces diffuse lower abdominal pain and nausea. There is exquisite tenderness over the hernia, which can usually be detected both by inspection and palpation of the hernial oriface. Failure to examine these areas is the most common cause for missing the diagnosis (Fig. 13).

Perforated sigmoid diverticulitis produces symptoms resembling appendicitis except that the pain is located in the left lower quadrant.

Acute salpingitis (pelvic inflammatory disease, or PID) produces diffuse, bilateral lower abdominal pain and fever. Motion of the cervix on vaginal and rectal examination produces marked pain, and there is diffuse tenderness of

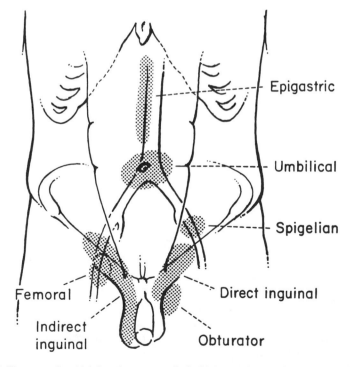

Figure 13. The areas in which hernias occur, all of which must be carefully examined in patients with abdominal pain. In addition to examining for the more common varieties of anterior hernias illustrated, one should always check for the less common perineal and lumbar hernias.

the pelvic structures. There may be a high fever, although patients with acute salpingitis do not appear very ill.

Mittelschmerz occurs in the middle of the menstrual cycle when the follicle ruptures. It usually occurs in young women and typically produces symptoms resembling acute appendicitis. There is generally no fever, and the symptoms subside after 6 to 12 hours of observation.

Obstruction of either the small intestine or colon produces crampy pain in the lower abdomen and around the umbilicus. As the disease progresses and the intestine becomes distended and ischemic, dull aching pain persists between the attacks of colic.

The presence of bacteria and white or red cells in the urinary sediment, together with the appropriate history, usually establishes the diagnosis of urinary tract disease. With a ureteral stone, pain is predictably intense and laterally located and commonly radiates from the kidney down to the pelvis, urethra, and inner thigh. Tenderness over the kidney may be noted. Delayed filling and then retention of contrast on the intravenous pyelogram confirms the diagnosis even if the stone itself is not visible.

The afflicted kidney, in acute pyelonephritis, is tender. There are associated high fever and chills and possibly rigors. The diagnosis can be confirmed through urinalysis and intravenous pyelogram.

Acute urinary retention can bring about severe pain and discomfort because of the distended bladder. A painful, tender midline mass below the umbilicus should always raise concern over this diagnosis. Always catheterize the bladder and then reevaluate the "mass."

Interpretation of Pain

An inflammatory process in one organ can induce strong symptoms from adjacent organs. For example, if an inflamed appendix is situated against the ureter or bladder, urinary symptoms may dominate the complaints. Other inflammatory conditions within the pelvis may also cause urinary tract symptoms.

Pain is an expression of both anatomic and physiologic factors. For example, the development of acute cholecystitis may commence with abrupt epigastric pain and nausea following a meal. Radiation of the pain to the right shoulder and flank may lead to a diagnosis of biliary colic and an attempt by the patient to pass a stone. After several hours, the pain may change to a constant, boring localized right upper quadrant pain, now suggesting a stone is lodged in the cystic duct, ie, acute cholecystitis. This obstruction may cause dilation of the gallbladder wall with compromise of its blood supply and ultimately necrosis of the organ's wall, resulting in gangrenous cholecystitis or even perforation and bile peritonitis.

Intermittent pain with a prolonged free interval indicates mechanical obstruction in the distal intestine. Intermittent pain with short free intervals also indicates obstruction but situated more proximally. Thus, the longer the pain-free interval, the more distal the obstruction is. If the character of the pain turns constant, blood supply to the intestine may be compromised and operation should not be delayed.

In summary, skillful interpretation of the pain and knowledge of pain patterns usually offer excellent clues to the diagnosis and indicate the site of the disease process and the dynamic changes that are occurring. Interpreting the pain and the associated information is the assemblage of the "pieces" that leads to the clinical solution of the pain "puzzle."

VOMITING

Vomiting is a common symptom of acute abdominal disease. Sometimes it is the only symptom of a life-threatening illness. The quantity and quality of the emesis are of great value in the differential diagnosis. In addition, the relationship of the onset of vomiting to the abdominal pain should be noted. For example, pain and vomiting occur almost simultaneously with the cystic duct obstruction of acute cholecystitis. With appendicitis, however, the anorexia and epigastric pain usually occur before the vomiting. An ileal adhesive small-intestinal obstruction will often produce pain many hours before the reflex vomiting. Vomiting results from one or more of the following causes:

1. Localized inflammation of the peritoneum or an intra-abdominal viscus with resultant reflex vomiting.
2. Obstruction (mechanical or paralytic) in the gastrointestinal tract or any hollow viscus (eg, bile duct, ureter).
3. Irritation of the central nervous system.

Reflex Vomiting

This type of vomiting occurs early in the development of acute abdominal disease, often simultaneously with the onset of pain. There may be a single episode or it can be protracted with retching. Vomitus usually consists of gastric contents with some bile. With severe renal or biliary colic, pancreatitis, or strangulation of a viscus, frequent vomiting is characteristic. With repeated vomiting, the content and appearance of the vomited material becomes more bilious. In pancreatitis, vomiting may be protracted and ultimately result in retching without production of vomitus. With appendicitis, salpingitis, and the milder forms of biliary colic, single episodes of vomiting are more typical. Sometimes there is no vomiting and the patient experiences only nausea and anorexia, both of which are often initial symptoms of disease causing peritonitis. In children, unexplained anorexia, nausea, or vomiting are signs requiring strict attention, since they may be the first clue in appendicitis.

Vomiting Appearing After Obstruction

The character of the vomitus in gastrointestinal tract obstruction varies in appearance and odor, depending on the location of the obstruction, and may give anatomic clues as to the site of the problem. Nonbilious vomiting implies obstruction proximal to the pylorus. Vomiting can be of large quantity, occur precipitously, and be projectile (pyloric stenosis) or occur as periodic, small regurgitations. Vomiting of food remnants that are not mixed with gastric juice indicates an obstruction in the esophagus.

With obstruction in the small intestine, the vomitus initially is more gastric in content but then gradually becomes bilious. After several hours, the vomitus acquires a feculant character, especially with low small-intestinal obstruction. Feculant vomiting indicates either mechanical obstruction or advanced paralytic ileus. The only exception to this rule is vomiting in the presence of a gastrocolic fistula.

In colonic obstruction, vomiting is a late symptom unless the cause is a volvulus. With volvulus, reflex vomiting occurs early and then gradually becomes more feculant in nature. With other causes of colonic obstruction, pain, distention, and changes in bowel habits dominate the clinical picture, and vomiting may not occur at all. Vomiting results not only from obstruction of the intestine but also from acute obstruction of a ureter or torsion of an ovarian pedicle. Therefore, any luminal structure that becomes acutely obstructed, regardless of the cause, can produce vomiting.

Vomiting is the major symptom in acute gastric dilatation. The copious vomiting resembles feculant vomiting in color but not in odor. In this situation there may be no anatomic obstruction but rather dysfunction of emptying related to surgical intervention, diabetes, or some diffuse infiltrating process like carcinoma or lymphoma.

Vomiting may also occur secondary to central nervous system irritation. A space-occupying lesion within the brain or a headache can result in emesis. Certain drugs, especially narcotics taken for the first time, may stimulate the vomiting center in the medulla.

The occurrence of vomiting varies sufficiently that its absence should not dissuade the examining physician from suspecting surgical disease in the presence of other significant abdominal findings. Likewise, the absence of vomiting should not discourage the surgeon from operating in a timely fashion when conditions otherwise indicate it.

ABNORMALITIES IN INTESTINAL FUNCTION

Many conditions causing pain in the abdomen are accompanied by a reduction in effective propulsive intestinal motility, which may progress to complete intestinal paresis or an increase in the frequency and volume of stool. Rather than merely asking if the patient is constipated or has diarrhea, it is more appropriate to ascertain what constitutes normal bowel function for this patient. Failure to pass flatus is a typical finding in mechanical obstruction. It should be noted, however, that even with complete obstruction, passage of gas may occur for the first 5 to 6 hours as air distal to the obstruction is evacuated.

Constipation that has lasted for several days is a common cause of abdominal pain and distention. A fecal impaction may also be a cause of obstruction.

Diarrhea is a common sign of enteritis and colitis but may also occur with appendicitis, ectopic pregnancy, salpingitis, and similar diseases that produce irritation of the rectum or sigmoid. Paradoxic diarrhea occurs with incomplete obstruction of the distal colon, typically by carcinoma or a fecal impaction. Mucus in the stool implies inflammation or tumor near the rectum or sigmoid colon (ulcerative colitis, pelvic abscess, intussusception, rectal carcinoma). Tenesmus, a repeated desire to evacuate the rectum, should clue the examiner to such conditions as pelvic abscess, ectopic pregnancy, appendicitis, salpingitis, or carcinoma.

Bloody diarrhea occurs with ulcerative colitis, diverticulitis, angiodysplasia, bacterial gastroenteritis, or colonic carcinoma. Massive hemorrhage in the proximal gastrointestinal tract resulting from ulcers, tumors, portal hypertension, or Meckel's diverticulum may also be included in the differential diagnosis of hematochezia. Finally, the passage of mucus and blood via the rectum is a late sign in intussusception or mesenteric infarction.

Bloating or distention can occur with many abdominal diseases and always occurs in advanced peritonitis. Abruptly appearing, marked abdominal distention occurs with volvulus, severe pancreatitis, and acute portal vein thrombosis and its associated ascites. Less abruptly appearing but eventually marked distention occurs with colon obstruction. Minimal to moderate distention with a tympanitic percussion sound is characteristic of mechanical small-intestinal obstruction, especially at the early stages, while moderate distention with a more sonorous percussion tone reflects paralytic ileus and occurs eventually with most inflammatory conditions in the abdomen.

UROGENITAL SYMPTOMS

Symptoms arising in the urinary tract are usually signs of disease of the urogenital organs but may also be indicative of disease in other abdominal organs. If the urine is bright-yellow or brownish, it may indicate jaundice. Red-tinged or smoky urine will appear in cases of hematuria or myonecrosis.

Urinary frequency can occur with appendicitis, ectopic pregnancy, salpingitis, urinary tract infection, ureteral stones, bladder or prostatic tumors, or urethral strictures. Nocturnal frequency should raise concerns over prostatitic hypertrophy. Urinary frequency more prominent during the day is commonly noted with urethral stricture. Intense dysuria is noted in cystitis but also occurs with urethritis or seminal vesiculitis.

Urinary retention developing either acutely or with a background of more chronic symptoms (difficulty or urinary hesitancy, diminished stream, dribbling, after drop) is usually the result of mechanical obstruction to emptying of the bladder. Acute urinary retention also occurs in patients influenced by alcohol, narcotics, or anticholinergic drugs. Postoperative patients, especially those undergoing anorectal manipulation, are prone to develop acute urinary retention. Pronounced distention of the bladder can give rise to severe abdominal pain, suggesting the possibility of an intestinal obstruction or even peritonitis.

With acute abdominal pain, macroscopic or gross hematuria occurs as a sign of urinary calculus, contusion or rupture of the urinary passages, tumor with hemorrhage, renal infarct, or necrotizing papillitis. The absence of hematuria does not exclude renal or ureteral stone as a cause of the acute abdominal pain, since blood may not pass if the stone completely obstructs the involved ureter.

Microscopic hematuria may be a sign of primary urinary tract disease but also occurs secondarily. Examples of this include appendicitis, in which the inflamed organ rests upon the bladder or ureter, or pelvic abscess, which produces similar reactions. In most instances, abdominal pain and hematuria mandate an intravenous pyelogram. Emergency cystoscopy and retrograde urography may also be indicated in some patients.

White cells in the urine indicate an inflammatory process in the urinary tract. If the pyuria is accompanied by bacteriuria, the presence of a urinary tract infection is likely. An increase of pyuria after prostatic massage supports a diagnosis of prostatitis.

Pregnancy and its related complications play an important role in the differential diagnosis of acute abdominal pain in women during their reproductive years. Any irregularity in the menstrual cycle should always be noted. Information as to whether menstruation is usually painful is a valuable clue in making a diagnosis of endometriosis. If syncope has occurred along with amenorrhea or "spotting," an ectopic pregnancy can be suspected. If the abdominal pain occurs at the halfway point between two cycles, a follicular rupture with hemorrhage (mittelschmerz) is likely. PID usually commences during or immediately after menstruation. Even if menstrual disturbances and abdominal pains are thought to be caused by complications of pregnancy or a female genital disease, it must be remembered that menstrual disturbances often occur quite independently of and simultaneously with diseases of other organs that cause peritonitis.

CHAPTER 2

■

The Physical Examination of the Abdomen

Joseph M. Vitello, MD, and Lloyd M. Nyhus, MD

The physical examination should *always* be preceded by a thorough and meaningful historical account of the patient's problem. Once this is obtained, the examiner may proceed. Too often, probing hands begin abdominal palpation without direction, which is much like hopping in a car and driving away without directions to one's destination. Although it is the abdomen that becomes the chief focus of attention in patients complaining of abdominal pain, the examiner must not overlook subtle information that may be gleaned from the rest of the physical examination.

INSPECTION

Inspection, the first step in the examination, should include not only the abdomen but also the general appearance of the patient. Really *look* at the patient! What is the influence of pain on him or her? Take note of the patient's activity as you approach. Is the patient talking jovially on the telephone or comfortably watching television, or does he or she appear ill? What position does the patient assume while in bed? The posture may be of value in the differential diagnosis and in some circumstances be diagnostic. Is the patient relaxed with an unaffected demeanor, or is he or she curled up and moaning, or writhing and crying out? Is the patient lying with the right leg flexed at the hip and knee because of psoas irritation? Observe the respiratory pattern and rate. Cyanosis and dyspnea do not necessarily arise from primary cardiac or pulmonary disease only. With peritonitis, breathing may be shallow and restricted to avoid painful movement of the abdominal wall. For this reason, respirations may become thoracic in character. There will be a compensatory increase in rate to maintain minute volume. For this reason a respiratory alkalosis often precedes the metabolic acidosis of sepsis. The patient with advanced peritonitis appears extremely ill, dehydrated, and anxious.

Observe the patient's face before and during the abdominal examination. A patient who smiles, giggles, or laughs during palpation of the abdomen is unlikely to have an urgent surgical problem and will benefit from a follow-up examination.

The patient's movements often give clues to the character of the pain. A patient with a perforated viscus and peritonitis will lie quietly in bed, but a patient with a mechanical intestinal obstruction will twist about and look uncomfortable during spasms of pain. Renal colic is a severe pain that does not allow the patient to be comfortable, regardless of position. Ischemic pain from intestinal infarction creates a distinctive complaint of pain out of proportion to the physical findings and a patient who rolls about on the bed. With acute pancreatitis, the individual often prefers to lie in the fetal position in an attempt to diminish pressure in the retroperitoneum. Asking a patient to rise out of bed and walk across the room can be revealing. The patient with localized peritonitis caused by appendicitis gets up gingerly, holds the right lower quadrant, and walks slowly with a scoliosis to the right to minimize lower abdominal pain.

The appearance of jaundice within the first few hours after the onset of pain can be difficult to judge on clinical examination, but this does occur with choledocholithiasis, cholangitis, pancreatitis, and sometimes with cholecystitis. The frenulum of the tongue examined in bright light will reveal jaundice before it is detected in the sclera.

TEMPERATURE

In the early course of acute abdominal disease, fever seldom occurs. The temperature should be measured rectally, by tympanic membrane, or through the pulmonary artery catheter. Oral temperatures are acceptable but less reliable. Axillary temperatures are not worth the effort and should be abolished. Many patients' normal temperatures fall below the 98.6°F cutoff, and therefore fevers of 99°F are potentially significant and should not be recorded as "afebrile." A rising temperature can accompany any inflammatory reaction but is a relatively late sign. Up to the moment of perforation, gangrenous appendicitis produces only a very modest rise in temperature. An elevated temperature is not always synonymous with bacterial infection. Rigors associated with fever suggest bacteremia and should prompt obtaining blood cultures and thorough searching for the source. The temperature may be helpful in the differential diagnosis. For example, it is unusual to see a high fever concomitant with the early pain of appendicitis. A marked febrile response, over 102°F

(38.9°C), is typical of bacterial peritonitis, salpingitis, pyelonephritis, and pneumonia. Spiking temperatures at the same time each day in a picket-fence pattern are seen with intra-abdominal abscess. In general, in the presence of abdominal pain, the higher the fever, the more serious is the intra-abdominal disease. Recall, however, that fever and abdominal pain do not always imply a condition requiring surgery (eg, familial Mediterranean fever). However, the variability in febrile response to peritoneal disease is so great that care must be taken not to include or exclude a diagnosis entirely on the basis of the temperature. The dehydrated or elderly patient may not express a febrile response to inflammatory disease, whereas the young child may have a high fever with a trivial problem. Hypothermia should also be noted, since it may be a more grave prognostication than fever in the septic patient. Use of an antipyretic should be avoided until the source of the fever can be identified, unless there are compelling reasons to suppress the temperature.

PULSE

Changes in the pulse rate are seldom noted in the early phase of abdominal disease. A patient with a gangrenous appendix may continue to have a normal pulse, even with marked local muscular spasm and pain. Noting the pulse may be of some value in following the progression of acute abdominal disease but when normal should not exclude the consideration of serious disease. A rising pulse rate, noted over the course of time and while performing repeated abdominal examinations, is a worrisome finding and should not be overlooked. Tachycardia is also a sign of hypovolemia or is commensurate with the degree of fever. Intra-abdominal hemorrhage is commonly associated with significant tachycardia before hypotension results. A pulse of 120 in a patient suffering blunt trauma to the abdomen should arouse suspicions of a significant injury and when the rate is 140 or greater, hypotension is not far away. Occasionally a very ill patient is noted to have no tachycardia. Be aware if the patient is on beta blockers or has atherosclerosis of the conduction system of the heart, in which case the pulse rate cannot elevate.

STEPS IN THE EXAMINATION OF THE ABDOMEN

Traditionally, the examiner stands on the right side of the patient; however, this is not essential. Use of improper technique in the art of abdominal examination and disregard for the patient's pain may result in an uncooperative and disgruntled patient, which may then make important serial examinations difficult and unrewarding. When observing a patient for the evolution of worsening abdominal pain, the same examiner should perform the repeat examination in the hope of detecting subtle changes. It is unnecessary to deeply and aggressively palpate the abdomen of a patient with florid peritonitis, since rebound tenderness can be elicited with a variety of more elegant maneuvers that are discussed below.

First, try to have the patient as relaxed as possible. The rapport developed during the history taking is most helpful and facilitates a reliable abdominal examination. A comfortable room temperature allows the patient to be exposed adequately without shivering and the resultant involuntary guarding. In addition, pay heed to the modesty of the patient by covering unnecessarily exposed areas. Children can be especially modest, and embarrassment may produce a shy, uncooperative patient, thereby complicating the abdominal examination.

Inspection

The inexperienced examiner will often begin with an almost unavoidable urge to palpate the abdomen and thus miss the visual clues that may be readily evident and meaningful. Inspection of the abdomen will immediately disclose any large hernias and can also reveal skin lesions or rashes that may be associated with painful symptoms, eg, herpes zoster. The number and location of abdominal scars may be helpful in the determination of the diagnosis. Any abdominal scar associated with crampy abdominal pain should raise the suspicion of an adhesive small-intestinal obstruction. In addition, the presence of a scar may help eliminate a likely cause of abdominal pain from the diagnosis. For example, the differential diagnosis of right lower quadrant abdominal pain may exclude appendicitis in the presence of a Pfannenstiel's incision performed for a hysterectomy and incidental appendectomy.

Observe whether the abdomen is scaphoid, distended, obese, or being held tense by the patient. The tense abdomen is under maximal muscular tension, a finding typical in acute perforated ulcer and chemical peritonitis (rigid abdomen). This type of finding may also be noted in the patient who has severe back pain, as with acute nucleus pulposus herniation, or the patient who voluntarily tenses in anticipation of a painful examination.

Distention of the abdomen is usually caused by dilated, gas- or fluid-filled intestine and is seen with both paralytic ileus and mechanical obstruction. Sometimes it may be difficult to differentiate an obese abdomen from a distended abdomen. Often the patient can be helpful in making this assessment: Is this your normal abdominal size or do you perceive distention? If the girth of the abdomen has developed over time, the patient may not observe this as readily but does usually note the need for larger size clothing or the need to let out belt notches. Distention of the abdomen is often serially measured with a tape measure to detect changes in size. We find this information of little help. A progressively developing ileus may distend the abdomen and not be of surgical significance. In addition, a large volume of fluid may be sequestered with little change in girth.

Take notice of engorged veins or an everted umbilicus, which raise the suspicion of ascites and liver disease. Visible peristalsis occurring during complaints of abdominal pain may be seen in the thin patient with an intestinal obstruction.

Cullen's sign occurs when there is bruising or ecchymosis at the umbilicus. This was first described in association with a ruptured ectopic pregnancy. Grey Turner's sign is a similiar discoloration in the flank, originally described with pancreatitis. While easy to detect, neither of these signs is specific, but generally they are clues to intra-abdominal or retroperitoneal hemorrhage.

Auscultation

Auscultation is the next phase of the abdominal examination. First, warm the chest piece of the stethoscope, since a cold instrument may create voluntary guarding in an adult and especially in the wary child. Many authors believe auscultation should be performed for 5 minutes before making an assessment of the bowel sounds. An absolute time constraint seems burdensome, and common sense should prevail. Sufficient time should be spent to assess absence or presence of bowel sounds. As in cardiac auscultation, once proficiency is obtained, the time spent listening and accurately interpreting the findings diminishes. Occasionally, special note is made of the presence or absence of bowel sounds in "all four quadrants." This has limited clinical relevance.

A truly "silent abdomen" has a distinct connotation to a surgeon and is noted in intra-abdominal catastrophes and with diffuse peritonitis. This is not a hard-and-fast rule, however. When present, the frequency and quality of the bowel sounds should be noted. Are they diminished, normal, or increased in frequency? It is possible to differentiate between mechanical obstruction and paralytic ileus by auscultation of the abdomen and noting the character of the bowel sounds. Early in the course of paralytic ileus (Fig. 14), bowel sounds may be decreased in frequency but are not absent. They are bubbling in character, reflecting the presence of accumulating gas and fluid within the intestine. The sounds may vary from low- to high-pitched tones. Later in an ileus, the bowel sounds are more markedly decreased in frequency, but rarely are they completely absent.

Early in the course of a mechanical obstruction, bowel sounds may be increased in frequency and occur concomitantly with the patient's report of cramping pain. High-pitched bowel sounds are compatible with either mechanical obstruction or resolving paralytic ileus. In mechanical obstruction, bowel sounds vary from medium- to very high-pitched, tend to be frequent, and to have a rushing or crescendo quality, whereas in paralytic ileus they are less frequent and have a more bubbling or tinkling quality, although the distinction between the two clinically is difficult. Later in the course of mechanical obstruction, as the bowel becomes fatigued, the repetitive pattern of the bowel sounds is lost and they are indistinguishable from those of paralytic ileus.

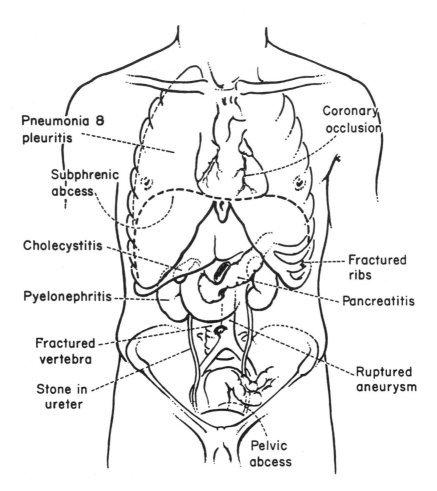

Figure 14. The common causes of paralytic ileus. Peritonitis from any source also causes paralytic ileus. Before an operation for intestinal obstruction is undertaken, it should be verified that the apparent obstruction is not simply a functional failure of peristalsis, secondary to some of the causes illustrated, which would not of itself require operative treatment.

In addition to mechanical obstruction, increased frequency and amplitude of bowel sounds (hyperperistalsis, borborygmi) are found in patients with gastroenteritis, upper gastrointestinal bleeding as a result of the cathartic effect of blood, and in the postprandial state. The sounds in these situations are of normal pitch but are frequent and may be continuous.

Hearing breath sounds or the heart while auscultating the abdomen

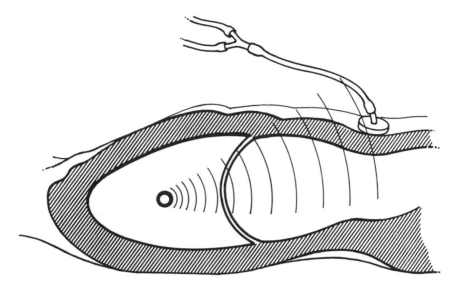

Figure 15. Breath sounds generated in the lungs can be heard through the anterior abdominal wall if the intestine is distended and fills the space between the diaphragm and the abdominal wall. This sign may be present with either paralytic ileus or mechanical obstruction but is more common with an ileus. The distention required is not great, and the phenomenon is also readily demonstrated after abdominal operations. As the ileus begins to resolve, breath sounds are no longer transmitted.

means that the entire space between the diaphragm and the anterior abdominal wall is occupied by loops of bowel (Fig. 15). The degree of distention required to produce this phenomenon is most characteristic of paralytic ileus but will be seen occasionally with distal small-intestine obstruction.

Auscultation of the abdomen may also detect bruits arising from turbulent flow in the renal or mesenteric arteries or an aortic aneurysm. Bruits or rubs heard over the liver may be noted with perihepatitis from pelvic inflammatory disease and hepatomas, but overall this is rare.

While auscultation is being performed, the application of steady downward pressure with the diaphragm of the stethoscope can be used as a form of abdominal palpation. This is mentioned for use in the malingering patient who complains of severe abdominal pain, especially with palpation, yet whose other findings are all normal. The distracted malingerer often fails to realize the examiner is doing more than just listening when performing this maneuver. This procedure can also be helpful with children to help localize maximal tenderness. Children with abdominal pain will often tense up when they are about to undergo palpation, making identification of localized abdominal pain difficult. Instead their attention can be distracted by "listening" and letting the stethoscope do the palpation.

Percussion

Percussion of the abdomen is the next step of the abdominal examination. This will help determine if abdominal distention is due to air (tympanitic) or fluid or a mass (dullness). Light percussion of the abdominal cavity can give valuable information concerning the distribution of gas and fluid. Dullness in the flanks, with a sonorous percussion tone over the central portions of the abdomen, is typical of free fluid in the abdominal cavity (Fig. 16). Large quantities of free fluid, as may occur in cirrhosis or carcinomatosis, may exhibit a percussion wave. If a large amount of free gas exists in the abdominal cavity, as may occur with a perforated colon or duodenal ulcer, there may be a sonorous percussion tone in those regions where dullness would normally exist, eg, over the liver (Fig. 17).

The liver and spleen, as well as any abdominal masses, should be percussed to determine their span and size.

The abdomen may also be distended by ascitic fluid or blood. Percussion of the patient in various positions to demonstrate shifting dullness usually indicates that the apparent distention is a result of fluid in the abdomen that is outside the intestine (Fig. 16B). Finally, percussion is a much more subtle and elegant way to detect peritonitis than direct palpation and sudden release. In appendicitis with localized parietal peritoneal irritation, percussion over the inflamed organ will produce rebound tenderness without the need to cause unnecessary discomfort to the patient. Likewise, percussion in the left lower quadrant will often produce a Rovsing's sign, with referral of maximal pain to the right lower quadrant. These maneuvers should virtually replace the antiquated method of heavy-handed deep palpation and sudden withdrawl of the examining hand to elicit "rebound tenderness." This latter maneuver may elicit a surprise reaction from the patient that is unrelated to the presence of peritoneal irritation and thus cause overestimation of the true incidence of peritonitis.

Palpation

Palpation is the last step in a thorough examination of the abdomen. Before we palpate, we ask the patient to cough vigorously. Characteristically, a patient with florid peritonitis declines or coughs weakly while holding his or her abdomen. As if by accident, we bump the bed or cart with a leg to transmit vibratory impulses to the patient in an attempt to elicit rebound tenderness. With performance of these maneuvers, peritonitis can easily be detected without even placing a hand on the patient! In addition, the malingerer is often unaware of these "tricks" and complains emphatically of pain with direct palpation yet produces no findings when asked to cough or the cart is jarred. A few final maneuvers that can be performed are to grasp the iliac crests and shake the patient or ask him or her to hop up and down, all in an attempt to detect subtle rebound tenderness.

Abdominal palpation is begun by asking the patient to point to the area where the pain began and is now located. It should be observed *how* the patient points to those areas. The patient who precisely points out maximal tenderness by placing one or two fingers directly over the affected area is demon-

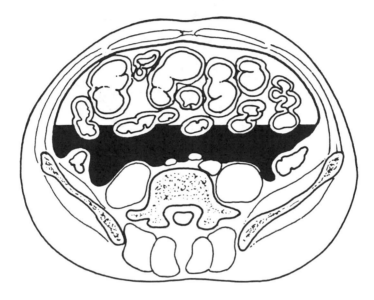

A

B

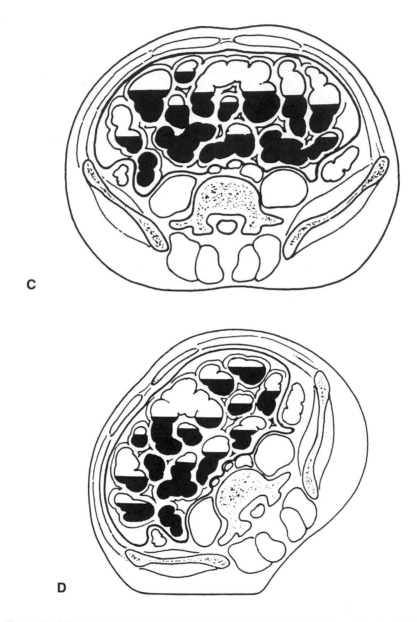

Figure 16. Differentiation of free fluid in the peritoneal cavity from fluid contained within loops of intestine. When there is free fluid (A), a level of dullness in the flank indicating the level of fluid in the peritoneal cavity can be identified easily by percussion. The patient is then tilted 45° on one side and the level of dullness again determined. With free fluid, the level of dullness shifts when the patient is turned on one side (B) (hence the term "shifting dullness"). If the fluid is contained within loops of bowel, the initial level of dullness determined by percussion in the flank is not sharply defined (C) and turning the patient to the side does not result in any marked change in the level of dullness (D).

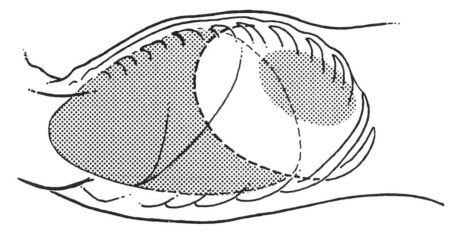

Figure 17. If there is a large amount of free air in the peritoneal cavity, normal dullness at percussion over the liver is lost and a sonorous or tympanitic note, similar to that of the lungs, is obtained. Tympany over the liver should always be sought in the midaxillary line. Tympany anteriorly is of no significance, since it may only be due to gas in the hepatic flexure of the colon or loops of small intestine.

strating localized peritoneal irritation. Diffuse pain is generally indicated with the entire hand placed or passed over the painful region in an ill-defined circular fashion. This is suggestive of visceral peritoneal pain.

Palpation should be carried out with warm hands, using flat fingers and the whole flat hand. Fingertip palpation alone is not enough. When palpation begins it is best to start in an area most remote from the perceived maximum tenderness, rather than to induce pain at the onset. Otherwise the patient, especially a child will become leery and not allow a more thorough examination in anticipation of being hurt.

Gentle palpation should be carried out first, moving gradually to the site where the patient complains of most intense pain. The hands must move gently, systematically, and methodically, with the fingers making small motions, as opposed to jumping around to various quadrants of the abdomen, since pain and tenderness may span more than one region. The pressure of the hands against the abdomen is increased slowly until the patient just feels tenderness or the muscles begin to become tense. It is not necessary to induce severe pain to evaluate an acute abdomen adequately. The degree of manual pressure required before the patient responds either verbally or with an increase of muscular tone is an excellent measure of involuntary guarding. Is the entire abdominal wall rigid, or boardlike? If so, is the guarding involuntary or voluntary? Voluntary guarding will diminish momentarily during expiration, so the patient should be asked to take a deep breath and then exhale while the examiner continues to palpate the abdomen. If the rigidity persists, the guarding is involuntary; the patient has peritonitis. Alternatively, the patient who is ticklish or voluntarily guards should be asked to flex both hips and bend both knees up as this will allow the recti to relax somewhat and facilitate the examination. If the entire abdomen is not rigid, localized areas of muscular spasm and tenderness must be sought. Palpation of the abdomen carried out with both hands will detect subtle differences of muscular tone between the left and right sides and between the upper and lower abdomen. Unilateral involuntary guarding cannot be done consciously and therefore implies an underlying inflammatory process.

Deeper palpation for the detection of abdominal masses or to elicit more deep-seated pain should be reserved for last and only in the patient who does not demonstrate peritonitis on the previous part of the examination. During this phase of the physical examination, attempts should be made to document hepatosplenomegaly, aortic abdominal aneurysm, or significant masses. The examiner should beware of those normal structures in the abdomen that may mimic an abnormal mass (Fig. 18).

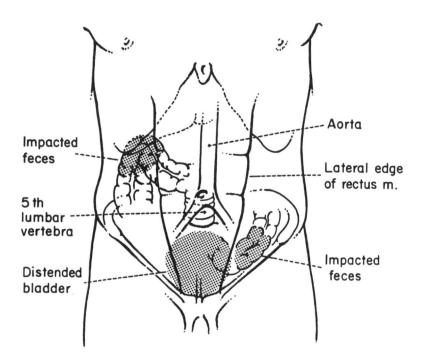

Figure 18. The common sources of error in palpating abdominal masses. The examiner must be sure that an apparent intra-abdominal mass is not, in fact, one of these normal structures. A pregnant uterus also is palpable in the mid lower abdomen. Lumbar vertebrae are easily palpated in thin, lordotic women.

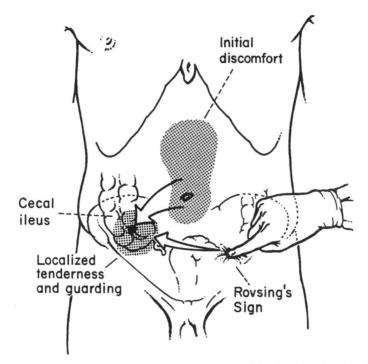

Figure 19. Demonstration of Rovsing's sign in association with other typical manifestations of acute appendicitis.

Pain produced by palpation may be of two types: direct, local tenderness, in which the pain is felt directly under the palpated area, and indirect or referred tenderness, in which the pain is experienced in an area other than the one being palpated. With appendicitis, for example, pain may be experienced over McBurney's point when palpation is performed in the left iliac fossa. This finding, called Rovsing's sign (Fig. 19), is a definite indication of peritoneal irritation. Comparative palpation of the muscular wall when it is relaxed and when it is tense can be carried out by having the patient lift his or her head from the pillow. Holding the head up keeps the abdominal muscles tense. If the source of the tenderness is within the anterior abdominal wall or involves the parietal peritoneum, pain will often be increased by tensing the muscles. If the source of tenderness is retroperitoneal or within the peritoneal cavity but does not involve the anterior parietal peritoneum or abdominal wall, usually no increase in pain is brought about by holding the head off the pillow.

The classic test to detect "rebound" tenderness is performed by palpating deeply and suddenly letting go. More intense pain produced when the peritoneum snaps back is a sign of parietal peritonitis. As already mentioned, this time-honored test for rebound tenderness is barbaric and will cause over-estimation of true rebound, especially in children. The more subtle maneuvers previously discussed are now employed to detect localized parietal peritoneal irritation and inflammation.

Hyperesthesias of the abdominal wall are noted in some conditions. This is classically described with appendicitis. When the skin is pinched or stroked with a pin, an exaggerated painful response occurs. This is an interesting clinical finding, but it is not to be relied upon to make the diagnosis of appendicitis or any other intra-abdominal condition. The pain elicited typically follows a dermatomal pattern.

Part of the abdominal examination should include a "punch" to the kidneys or the flanks to assess the degree of tenderness in this area. Not uncommonly, pyelonephritis or kidney stones can present with anterior abdominal pain; however, detailed examination reveals maximal tenderness is detected in the costovertebral angle.

In doubtful clinical situations, one examination may not be enough. Repeated abdominal palpation by the same examiner employing the same technique is important in correctly evaluating the patient with abdominal pain and disease in evolution.

Other Helpful Maneuvers

Psoas Sign. The patient lying supine is asked to attempt to raise a straight leg against the pressure of the examiner's hand on his or her shin (Fig. 20). Pain will result if an inflammatory process (eg, appendicitis) involves or lies

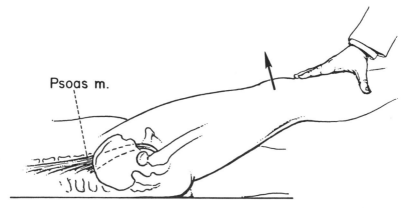

Psoas m.

Figure 20. The psoas sign. Raising a straight leg against resistance or, alternatively, passive hyperextension of the thigh posteriorly moves the psoas muscle. If there is an inflammatory process in contact with the psoas muscle, pain results from this maneuver.

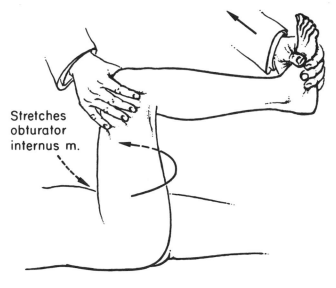

Stretches obturator internus m.

Internal rotation of flexed thigh

Figure 21. The obturator sign. If there is a pelvic inflammatory process in contact with the obturator internus muscle, passive internal rotation of the hip results in pain.

near the psoas muscle or if an acute primary disease process (eg, herniated nucleus pulposus) involves the lumbosacral spine.

Obturator Sign. With the patient supine, the hip and knee are each flexed to 90° and the leg then rotated (Fig. 21). Pain will result if an inflammatory process (pelvic abscess, appendicitis, salpingitis) involves or lies near the obturator internus muscle.

Murphy's Sign. The flat hand is held below the right costal margin, applying moderate pressure to the subcostal area. The patient is asked to take a deep breath. A positive test occurs when tenderness and pain occur as the liver or gallbladder descends against the palpating hand. The patient stops breathing in midinspiration. This sign is classically described with acute cholecystitis but may also be noted in patients with hepatitis, space-occupying lesions of the liver, and pleuritis.

Kehr's Sign. Kehr's sign occurs when the upper quadrants are being palpated and the patient complains of pain at the top of the shoulder. This is classically described on the left side and associated with an injured spleen. The pathophysiology relates to the C4 innervation of the diaphragm and referred pain. The sign can occur on the right side also. Diaphragmatic irritation from any source may produce a positive Kehr's sign. The sign may also be elicited by placing a patient in Trendelenburg position and assessing shoulder or neck pain.

Rectal Examination. This procedure, though usually done as the last part of the physical examination, must not be omitted in any patient complaining of abdominal pain. On occasion it may yield the only positive findings of the entire examination. Rectal palpation is always of importance because inflammatory lesions in the abdomen may be shielded by intestine and omentum and not involve the anterior parietal peritoneum. No signs may then be apparent on examination of the anterior abdominal wall. It is only with rectal and vaginal examination that such inflammatory lesions may be detected and information concerning accumulation of exudate, blood, or pus in the pelvic cavity uncovered.

The rectal examination can be distressing to the patient. In order to avoid discomfort, palpation should be carried out with a well-lubricated, gloved finger. Insert the finger slowly, allowing time for the sphincter to relax. If the finger is introduced too roughly or quickly, there may result spasm and pain of such severity as to mask true pelvic tenderness. After the finger is introduced and the fingertip lies free in the lumen of the rectum, wait a few sec-

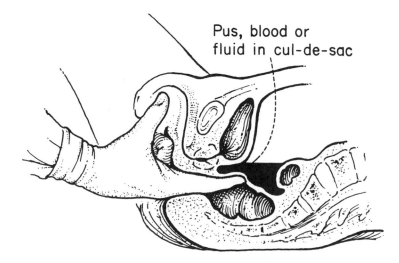

Pus, blood or
fluid in cul-de-sac

Figure 22. Pus, blood, or fluid in the pelvis collects in the pouch of Doug-las (cul-de-sac) and can be palpated on rectal examination.

onds to give the patient time to become accustomed to the sensation of anal dilation before further examination is begun. Palpation directed posteriorly against the hollow of the sacrum should be the first step in digital exploration of the rectum. There is rarely any disease in this area, so that palpation here establishes a base line, reflecting the patient's general discomfort associated with rectal examination. Tenderness, reflecting the presence of pathologic lesions in other areas, will then be more apparent. Tenderness in the pouch of Douglas can be ascertained when the examining finger is carried anteriorly; if inflammation exists, the patient complains of pain. Fluctuation here makes the diagnosis of a pelvic abscess almost certain (Fig. 22).

The rectal examination also reveals the condition of the prostate and seminal vesicles, as well as the possible presence of a tumor in the rectum. Finally, the gloved finger is removed, and any stool procured should be tested for the presence of occult blood. Vaginal examination provides information on the condition of the uterus and fallopian tubes. Pain elicited by motion of the

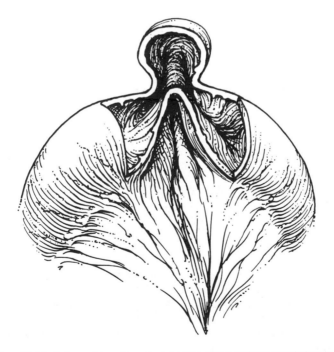

Figure 23. In a Richter's type of hernia, only a portion of the antimesenteric border of the intestine is involved in the hernia. As the hernia enlarges, more of the intestine is drawn into the hernia sac, eventually kinking the intestine and producing obstruction. Strangulation of the herniated intestinal wall can occur at any time.

cervix is suggestive evidence that the pelvic tissues around the uterus are inflamed (PID).

Palpation of Hernial Openings. In every instance of abdominal pain, the hernial openings should be carefully palpated (Fig. 13). Direct and indirect inguinal hernias should pose no diagnostic difficulties. Although a small hernia in the femoral canal is sometimes difficult to diagnose, a larger hernia is usually detectable by palpation if one remembers to examine this area. In the obese patient, a hernia may be more difficult to detect, especially if a large pannus exists. Hernias that produce signs and symptoms of an acute abdomen must be obstructed or strangulated or both. The herniated mass will be tender to palpation. A Richter's hernia (Fig. 23) is particularly difficult to palpate and often overlooked or missed during a cursory examination. It is usually demonstrated only when peritoneal irritation resulting from actual or threatening perforation has occurred.

REPEAT EXAMINATION UNDER ANESTHESIA

If the abdominal findings, laboratory evaluation, and clinical picture are consistent and operation is indicated, a golden opportunity exists to repeat the examination of the abdomen once general anesthesia has been induced. Muscular spasm will now be reduced or absent and voluntary guarding eliminated. A mass that could not be felt with the patient awake may now be clearly appreciated. This may help confirm the clinical impression or redirect the location of an abdominal incision.

SUGGESTED READING

Bates B. *A Guide to Physical Examination and History Taking.* 5th ed. Philadelphia, PA: JB Lippincott Co; 1990.

DeGowin and DeGowin's Bedside Diagnostic Examination. 5th ed. New York, NY: Macmillan Inc; 1987.

Guckian JC. *The Clinical Interview and Physical Examination.* Philadelphia, PA: JB Lippincott Co; 1987.

Macleod J, Munro J. *Clinical Examination: A Textbook for Students and Doctors.* 7th ed. New York, NY: Churchill Livingstone Inc; 1986.

Sapira JD. *The Art and Science of Bedside Diagnosis.* Baltimore, MD: Urban and Schwarzenberg Inc; 1990.

Wiener SL. *Differential Diagnosis of Acute Pain by Body Region.* New York, NY: McGraw-Hill Book Co; 1993.

CHAPTER 3

■

Laparoscopy as an Aid to Diagnosis

Joseph M. Vitello, MD

Laparoscopy is the endoscopic visualization of the intraperitoneal contents. In most situations this is accomplished by first establishing a pneumoperitoneum through the insufflation of carbon dioxide into the peritoneal cavity. Laparoscopy, while an invasive procedure, has recently gained new appreciation as a diagnostic tool for the general surgeon and as an aid to the rapid diagnosis of abdominal disorders. Laparoscopy has also become an important therapeutic tool. However, the focus of this chapter is on its diagnostic use.

Inspection of the intraperitoneal structures is a valuable adjunct to physical examination and biochemical and radiologic testing. In previous eras, when the diagnosis remained in question despite extensive testing, the exploratory laparotomy was referred to as the ultimate diagnostic "test." Recently, resurgence in the use of laparoscopy by the general surgeon has changed this attitude and made direct inspection of the abdominal organs a common procedure.

The concept of visualizing internal organs is not a new one. Abulkanim, an Arabian physician in the 8th century used a deflected mirror and light source to view the cervix and vaginal canal. In 1901, Kelling used the term "celioscopy" when he employed a cystoscope to examine the peritoneal contents of a dog. Jacobaeus, in 1910, used this technique for the first time on a human. These initial endeavors, while primitive, represent the birth of modern-day laparoscopy. An explosion of technology has improved optical systems, video has been added so all may view the procedure, and instrumentation has advanced concomitantly.

Most laparoscopy is performed in an operating room with the aid of general anesthesia, although this is not mandatory. There are reports of the performance of laparoscopy with local and epidural anesthesia. Laparoscopy is a two-part technique. First is the production of the pneumoperitoneum and insertion of the various trocars; second is visualization and manipulation of the intra-abdominal structures.

THE TECHNIQUE

Production of an adequate pneumoperitoneum and safe introduction of the trocars is essential. A variety of techniques exist. The percutaneous method, in which a Veress needle for insufflation of the carbon dioxide is blindly introduced into the peritoneal cavity, is quick, relatively easily learned, and has a low incidence of problems in experienced hands. However, a variety of complications have been reported, most commonly, impalement of a solid or hollow organ or vessel. For this reason, I favor the open method (Hasson technique), in which a small periumbilical incision is made. Subsequently the fascia and peritoneum are opened under direct vision and the trocar used for the introduction of the laparoscope is then placed into the peritoneal cavity under direct vision. This method avoids all the theoretical complications associated with the blind percutaneous introduction of the insufflating needle and trocar.

The second part of laparoscopy is visualization and manipulation of the intra-abdominal structures. This requires skills learned through working with experienced laparoscopists and laboratory-honed practice with animal or lifelike models.

Laparoscopy should not be—nor was it intended to be—a substitute for a thorough history and complete physical examination or a replacement for good clinical judgment. There is, however, a subset of patients for whom the history is unobtainable or inaccurate, the physical examination is unreliable or equivocal, or routine radiologic testing becomes cumbersome. Patients who fit into any of these categories may benefit from the use of laparoscopy as an extension of the physical examination.

Because laparoscopy is an expensive and invasive technique, with potential complications and even possible mortality, it should be employed according to the needs of the patient and the physician in the particular clinical situation. However, because diagnostic laparoscopy has been shown in several large series to have less than a 2% complication rate, hesitancy in the use of this technique is unwarranted.

INDICATIONS

The indications for the use of laparoscopy as an extension of the physical examination are listed in Table 7. In these conditions, the findings of a physical examination alone may be equivocal. Delay may be ill-advised or hazardous.

TABLE 7. USES OF DIAGNOSTIC LAPAROSCOPY IN GENERAL SURGERY

Assessment of blunt or penetrating trauma to the thoracoabdominal or abdominal cavity
Evaluation of acute abdominal pain
Evaluation of subacute peritoneal conditions
Evaluation of chronic abdominal pain
Staging of intra-abdominal malignant tumors
Liver biopsy
Evaluation of the critically ill patient with occult sepsis or abdominal pain

Blunt or Penetrating Trauma

The use of laparoscopy in the setting of blunt or penetrating trauma is not new; however, the current enthusiasm for this usage is. With blunt abdominal trauma, laparoscopy may be more definitive than diagnostic peritoneal lavage or computed tomography. Overlooking small-intestinal injury resulting from blunt trauma is a major pitfall with other diagnostic techniques; it may be more easily detected with laparoscopy. In the multiply traumatized patient who has major orthopedic or neurosurgical injuries, laparoscopy in the emergency department may allow earlier triage to the appropriate subspecialist without concern over missed abdominal injuries. In thoracoabdominal penetrating trauma, laparoscopy can be used to identify peritoneal penetration and define the actual injury. Diaphragmatic involvement from stab wounds to the thoracoabdominal region can be difficult to detect and may be more readily seen with laparoscopy. Stab wounds to the upper abdomen resulting in liver laceration often have ceased bleeding by the time laparotomy is performed. Perhaps laparoscopy has a role to play in these patients. Negative results from laparoscopy in cases of penetrating trauma may allow for less observation time and earlier discharge from the hospital or emergency department. Several studies are ongoing to identify laparoscopy's precise role in the presence of blunt and penetrating trauma.

Acute Abdominal Pain

Gynecologists have been performing laparoscopy quite proficiently and safely for years. But most general surgeons were never trained in laparoscopy. Historically, when a female patient presented with atypical lower abdominal pain and appendicitis seemed possible but uncertain, the general surgeon frequently called the gynecologist. The patient would be "scoped" to view the abdominal contents, specifically the pelvic organs. If a normal appendix was viewed, the general surgeon avoided an unnecessary appendectomy. If inflamed, the appendix would then be removed by the surgeon through a right lower quadrant (RLQ) incision.

The diagnostic dilemma of RLQ pain, especially in the female patient, is problematic for many physicians. It is well documented that the diagnostic error rate for appendicitis is highest in younger women, usually in their reproductive years, when other gynecologic causes may mimic appendicitis. The false-negative rate has approached 40% in some series. The list of differential diagnoses for RLQ pain is extensive, and many of the causes do not require surgical treatment. Many surgeons, not wanting to operate needlessly, adopt a wait-and-see policy. Others extend diagnostic procedures and expense with ultrasound, barium enema, computed tomography, and prolonged hospitalization and observation. Laparotomy is often performed for unexplained RLQ pain through a small incision. If the appendix is found to be normal, the incision is enlarged until the true source of the problem can be identified. Many conditions require no further surgery and the procedure is terminated. If the appendix shows no pathologic changes, the procedure is justified by the consequent false-negative appendectomy rate. Thus laparoscopy to evaluate the appendix and pelvic organs in this setting makes good sense. Its chief advantage is that it may save the patient a formal laparotomy if something of a nonsurgical nature is discovered. This should lead to more timely diagnosis and less delay in definitive treatment. Other presumed advantages include the ability to perform a more thorough evaluation of the total abdominal cavity, better cosmesis, less postoperative pain, less adhesion formation and wound infection, and quicker return to work and activities. For these reasons, a watch-and-wait plan for acute abdominal pain, especially RLQ pain, can be avoided. Several important questions that remain to be answered include the cost-benefit ratio for early laparoscopy versus serial laboratory evaluations and examinations.

When laparoscopy is performed for the evaluation of lower abdominal pain in the female patient, a uterine cannula introduced into the cervix allows for greater and easier mobilization of the uterus and subsequent visualization of pelvic structures. Catheterization of the urinary bladder should be performed so that distention of this organ will not interfere with the examination of the pelvic structures. In addition, the patient should be placed in slight lithotomy position to facilitate examination and aid in separating the small intestine from the pelvis. It has been stated that if this protocol is followed, the appendix may be seen in 90% to 97% of instances, but certainly this is operator-dependent.

Subacute Peritoneal Conditions

Certain subacute conditions are very difficult to diagnose clinically or based only on the history and physical examination. One example is tuberculous peritonitis. There is a recent increase in the prevalence of tuberculosis (TB), and intra-abdominal TB is on the rise. Not only can the diagnosis be strongly suspected in the presence of granulomas identified at laparoscopy, but tissue can be procured for definitive identification of the causative organism.

Chronic Abdominal Pain

On occasion a patient will complain of chronic abdominal pain. An extensive evaluation, using the examiner's skills along with adjunctive laboratory and radiologic testing, may be inconclusive. In this setting there are numerous success stories written about the value of diagnostic laparoscopy for the evaluation of obscure abdominal pain. A laparoscopy with negative results often leads to the belief that the cause of the pain is psychosomatic. In these chronic pain syndromes it may be more cost-effective to reach for the laparoscope early.

Adhesions are commonly blamed for chronic abdominal pain. Most physicians' training, experience, and beliefs teach that unless there is a component of intestinal obstruction, lysis of adhesions provides no benefit to a patient complaining of abdominal pain. Laparoscopy's role in this setting is to exclude other causes of abdominal pain. Therapeutically, lysis of adhesions can be performed through the laparoscope, occasionally with successful results. Whether this is the result of a placebo effect or anecdotal remains controversial.

Staging of Intra-abdominal Malignant Tumors

Despite the sophistication of modern diagnostic equipment, occasionally a patient undergoes an exploratory laparotomy and unsuspected carcinomatosis is detected. If intra-abdominal neoplasm is suspected but unproven, laparoscopy allows visualization to detect small metastases that were beyond the resolution of radiographic detection. Biopsy can easily be performed to obtain histopathologic confirmation.

The traditional approach to patients with periampullary and pancreatic carcinoma in the absence of obvious metastasis has been exploratory laparotomy. However, more often than not, at laparotomy the tumor is found to be metastatic or unresectable. The rationale for staging pancreatic cancer with the laparoscope is based on the concept that only 5% to 10% of pancreatic malignant tumors are resectable. Usually the diagnosis of adenocarcinoma of the pancreas can be achieved through percutaneous fine-needle aspiration under computerized tomography or ultrasound guidance. Furthermore, biliary stents will provide palliation from jaundice and pruritus at less cost, reduced morbidity, and shorter hospital stay than surgical bypasses. Therefore, many surgeons now advocate laparoscopy to aid in determination of metastasis before formal laparotomy. When previously unrecognized metastasis is encountered, the procedure is terminated with less operating room time and less pain and quicker recovery for the patient.

Liver Biopsy

The diagnosis of liver disease is not normally within the realm of the general surgeon. However, it often becomes necessary to obtain tissue to confirm a clinical suspicion as to the cause of liver abnormalities. The procurement of liver tissue should really be thought of as an extension of the physical examination of these patients. In high-risk patients for whom percutaneous biopsy may be hazardous, a laparoscopic directed biopsy may be safer. If a space-occupying lesion exists within the liver and other attempts at biopsy have proven unsuccessful or nondiagnostic, a laparoscopic assisted biopsy can be of value.

Evaluation of a Critically Ill Patient with Occult Sepsis or Abdominal Pain

Evaluation of abdominal pain in the patient under intensive care can be problematic. These patients are often too sick to undergo a negative laparotomy, yet many have intra-abdominal pathologic conditions in need of surgical treatment. Often these patients are intubated, and history is not obtainable. In the critically ill intensive care unit patient who develops abdominal pain or occult sepsis or is moribund, physical examination is of limited help. A plethora of monitoring lines and various intravenous drips and life-support systems can make patient transport for diagnostic testing cumbersome. Reluctance to move the patient leads to delay in diagnosis, which may increase the gravity of the condition and even the likelihood of death. Often the patients have borderline cardiac or renal function, which makes the use of intravenous contrast hazardous. Diagnostic laparoscopy in this setting may be an important tool and avoid nontherapeutic laparotomy or confirm the indications for exploration and definitive treatment. The laparoscopic procedure can often be performed in the intensive care unit, thereby avoiding the transportation difficulties.

CONTRAINDICATIONS

While laparoscopy has many theoretical advantages, it is not a panacea. Often, critically ill patients have marked abdominal distention with ileus. Initial trocar placement to produce the pneumoperitoneum can be difficult. Laparoscopic visualization may be limited, depending upon the degree of ileus. Contraindications to laparoscopy include uncorrected coagulopathy, peritonitis, known extensive adhesions ("frozen abdomen") since they preclude good visualization, and a contraindication to general anesthesia. The last contraindication prevails only to the extent that because the production of a pneumoperitoneum is quite uncomfortable for most patients, it is usually performed under general anesthesia. If inflating pressures are kept low, however, discomfort is as well, and the procedure can be accomplished with local anesthesia.

SUGGESTED READING

Brandt CP, Priebe PP, Eckhauser ML. Diagnostic laparoscopy in the intensive care patient. *Surg Endosc.* 1993; 7:168–172.

Easter DW, Cuschieri A, Nathanson LK, et al. The utility of diagnostic laparoscopy for abdominal disorders: audit of 120 patients. *Arch Surg.* 1992; 127:379–383.

Forde KA, Treat MR. The role of peritoneoscopy (laparoscopy) in the evaluation of the acute abdomen in critically ill patients. *Surg Endosc.* 1992; 6:219–221.

Nagy AG, James D. Diagnostic laparoscopy. *Am J Surg.* 1992; 157:490–493.

Nowzaradan Y, Westmoreland J, McCarver CT, et al. Laparoscopic appendectomy for acute appendicitis: indications and current use. *J Laparoendosc Surg.* 1991; 1:247–257.

Saye WB, Rives DA, Cochran EB. Laparoscopic appendectomy: three years' experience. *Surg Laparosc Endosc.* 1991; 1:109–115.

Warshaw AL, Gu Z, Wiitenberg J, et al. Preoperative staging and assessment of resectability of pancreatic cancer. *Arch Surg.* 1990; 125:230–233.

Whitworth CM, Whitworth PW, Sanfillipo J, et al. Value of diagnostic laparoscopy in young women with possible appendicitis. *Surg Gynecol Obstet.* 1988; 167:187–190.

Zucker KA, ed. *Surgical Laparoscopy.* St. Louis, Mo. Quality Medical Publishing; 1991.

CHAPTER 4

■

Emergency Ancillary Investigations

Mark A. Malangoni, MD
Christopher P. Brandt, MD

Because patients with acute abdominal pain urgently require a diagnosis, time-consuming investigations are not feasible. However, a variety of simple investigations are easy to perform and can help to establish the proper diagnosis. The usefulness of most of these diagnostic tests is based primarily on the demonstration of an abnormal finding or set of findings that should confirm what is suggested by the history and physical examination. A negative test in a patient with acute abdominal pain often does not provide any useful information; a negative test does not "rule out" anything. Test results that conflict with the clinical signs and symptoms should be viewed with suspicion, and the discrepancy should be clarified by further evaluation.

The expanse of available investigational radiographic procedures places an onus on the physician to be selective in choosing diagnostic tests on the basis of clinical suspicion. Failure to use testing efficiently within the time constraints imposed by the patient's acute condition can unnecessarily delay appropriate management. Although these studies are addressed singly here, in practice, it is imperative to integrate the results of all tests with the history and physical findings to achieve a diagnosis.

URINALYSIS

Examination of the urinary sediment and qualitative evaluation of the urine for abnormal excretory products is a test that can be done easily and with minimal equipment. A clean-catch sample or one obtained by catheterization is preferable. Urinalysis often provides more useful information than any other single test.

The presence of glucose in the urine indicates hyperglycemia that can be a manifestation of uncontrolled infection in a patient with diabetes. The presence of protein, bile, or ketones in the urine can indicate chronic renal disease, jaundice, and dehydration, respectively, but these abnormalities may not pinpoint the exact cause of acute abdominal pain. The urinary specific gravity usually reflects the patient's state of hydration. In many situations of acute abdominal pain, the specific gravity of the urine is high, reflecting the dehydration that accompanies serious illness. When this value is inappropriately low, it usually suggests the presence of chronic renal disease.

Microscopic pyuria of 5 to 20 white blood cells (WBCs) per high-power field (HPF) in the centrifuged sediment of an uncontaminated and properly obtained urine sample can represent an infectious or inflammatory process that is related either to the urinary tract or to adjacent intraperitoneal organs. More than 20 WBCs/HPF in a spun urine specimen strongly suggests a urinary tract infection. This diagnosis can be confirmed immediately if bacteria are seen on microscopic examination or Gram's stain of the urine sediment. Although urinary tract infections can occur when fewer than 20 WBCs/HPF are present in the spun urine, this lesser degree of pyuria also can be due to an inflammatory process near the bladder or ureter, such as appendicitis or a pelvic abscess. The presence of nitrate in the urine in the setting of pyuria suggests infection caused by a nitrate-producing organism such as *Proteus mirabilis.*

Gross or microscopic hematuria is always abnormal. Inflammatory processes close to the urinary tract are associated with microscopic hematuria of fewer than 30 red blood cells (RBCs) per HPF. More than 30 RBCs/HPF indicates disease of the urinary tract resulting from ureteral stones, tumors, trauma, or infection. When this degree of microscopic hematuria occurs, an intravenous pyelogram (IVP) should be done to confirm the cause and site of disease within the urinary tract.

Casts in the urinary sediment can indicate pyelonephritis (WBC casts), chronic renal disease, or glomerulonephritis (RBC casts). Although unusual, these disorders are frequently accompanied by abdominal pain. Granular casts indicate damage to the renal tubules.

BLOOD STUDIES

Blood Count

A decrease in hemoglobin and hematocrit values in the presence of abdominal pain may represent sequestered intra-abdominal or intraluminal hemorrhage. Rapid blood loss, as may occur with a ruptured ectopic pregnancy or ruptured subcapsular hematoma of the spleen may produce little change in the hematocrit or hemoglobin values until translocation of fluid from the extracellular or intracellular space or administration of intravenous (IV) fluids allows the hematocrit to decrease as the blood volume is replenished. Low

RBC indices suggest chronic blood loss that may be caused by a malignant tumor of the gastrointestinal (GI) tract as well as benign diseases that cause GI bleeding. Abdominal pain can occur after perforation of a gastroduodenal ulcer or tumor that has been a source of blood loss into the intestinal tract. The triad of trauma, cramping abdominal pain associated with acute GI bleeding, and the presence of a low hemoglobin value strongly suggests hematobilia.

The presence of an increased WBC count (leukocytosis) is a nonspecific finding in patients with acute abdominal pain and can be misleading. Leukocytosis can occur in response to any infection or inflammatory disease. Pregnancy, use of steroids, and the postsplenectomy state are other causes of an increased WBC count. Although many patients with acute abdominal pain have an increased total WBC count, there is considerable variability among individuals, and some patients with acute intra-abdominal infections have a normal total WBC count. Leukopenia also may be an important sign of infection, particularly in older patients and infants. Severe leukopenia is associated with a poor prognosis and can be associated with a less severe manifestation of abdominal pain.

The differential WBC count is often a more reliable indicator of infection than the total count. Most patients who have an abnormal total leukocyte count in response to an infection have an increased percentage of immature forms and WBC precursors in the differential count (shift to the left) represented by bands, myelocytes, and metamyelocytes. These WBC precursors are released from the bone marrow in response to infection. As an example of the usefulness of the differential WBC count, less than 5% of patients with appendicitis have both a normal total leukocyte count and normal differential count.

Examination of a peripheral blood smear not only provides an estimate of the granulocyte response but also may give additional useful information. Eosinophilia can indicate a parasitic infestation or an allergic reaction; patients who have viral infections or acute adrenal insufficiency may have lymphocytosis. Examination of RBCs in the peripheral smear may reveal the abnormalities of sickle cell disease or evidence of lead intoxication. These conditions can also be associated with acute abdominal pain. Although thrombocytopenia is rarely associated with abdominal pain, allergic purpuras are unusual causes of abdominal pain and are nearly always accompanied by thrombocytopenia.

Serum Chemistries

An elevation of the serum bilirubin level usually only confirms obvious clinical jaundice; however, subclinical hyperbilirubinemia can represent biliary tract infection or obstruction. At times, an increased total bilirubin level can reflect cholestasis associated with infections not directly involving the liver and biliary tree. A direct bilirubin component of more than 80% supports the diagnosis of biliary tract obstruction.

Serum aminotransferase (ALT and AST) levels are sensitive but nonspecific indicators of hepatocellular injury and are most helpful in identifying acute hepatocellular diseases such as hepatitis. Moderate elevations in ALT and AST levels may be seen in a number of conditions, such as hepatitis, alcoholic liver disease, cirrhosis, heart failure, acute cholecystitis, bile duct obstruction, and drug reactions. Elevations in aminotransferase levels also may be found in patients with severe injuries to the cardiac or skeletal muscle. Extreme elevations (more than eight to ten times normal) are associated with severe cellular injury. They are caused by acute hepatitis or toxic injury to the liver.

Alkaline phosphatase level is elevated in 75% of patients with prolonged cholestasis. However, this test does not distinguish between intrahepatic or extrahepatic obstruction. An isolated elevation of alkaline phosphatase level may occur in the presence of a partial bile duct obstruction, hepatic abscess, sarcoidosis, or metastatic carcinoma. Abnormalities of these serum chemistries may suggest, but rarely establish, a specific diagnosis.

Although serum electrolyte values can be abnormal in patients with abdominal pain, these alterations are usually the result of associated vomiting, diarrhea, or dehydration and do not indicate the cause of the abdominal pain. Hyperglycemia can occur in relation to the "stress" of an infection that causes abdominal pain, or it can indicate the presence of infection in a patient with diabetes who previously had well-controlled blood glucose values. An increased blood urea nitrogen (BUN) level frequently reflects dehydration. However, an elevated BUN or creatinine level can also be an indicator of renal failure associated with abdominal pain, most particularly acute glomerulonephritis.

Determination of Amylase Level

An elevated serum amylase level is often used to confirm the diagnosis of acute pancreatitis. In fact, when levels of pancreatic isoenzymes are determined, pancreatic amylase level is elevated in only two thirds of patients with clinical signs of acute pancreatitis. Elevation of nonpancreatic isoamylase levels in patients with acute abdominal pain may be related to inflammation at other sites of amylase production, such as the small intestine, salivary glands, genital tract, or liver. Chronic renal failure also can cause increases in serum amylase level because of impairment of clearance and excretion of this enzyme.

Because elevations in serum amylase level can be transient or can escape detection because of rapid glomerular filtration and excretion of this enzyme, measurement of urinary amylase has been proposed as a more accurate method to establish the diagnosis of acute pancreatitis. Determinations can be done on a single urine sample, but there is less variability when a specimen is collected over a 4- to 6-hour period. There is no conclusive study demonstrating that an elevation in urinary amylase level is a more sensitive indicator of pancreatitis. Therefore, this study is usually not of added benefit.

Determination of Human Chorionic Gonadotropin Level

Human chorionic gonadotropin (HCG) is a glycoprotein hormone secreted by trophoblastic tissue. A number of sensitive urine or serum assays exist for determination of HCG levels, and this test should be considered in any woman of child-bearing age who presents with acute abdominal pain. A sensitive qualitative assay can be easily and rapidly performed and is an appropriate screening test. A positive test confirms a pregnancy. More than 95% of women with ectopic pregnancies have a positive test. A quantitative radioimmunoassay for the beta (β) subunit of HCG is the most precise measurement available. A negative assay for β-HCG excludes pregnancy with greater than 99% predictive accuracy. A very small percentage of patients with an ectopic pregnancy have a negative HCG screening assay, but the quantitative test is elevated in this group of patients.

Determination of C-reactive Protein Level

C-reactive protein (CRP) is a constituent of plasma thought to represent a nonspecific indicator of acute inflammation. The level of CRP may be elevated in a number of clinical situations associated with abdominal pain. In 99% of healthy adults, the serum CRP concentration is normally less than 10 mg/L. The utility of CRP measurement in abdominal pain has been studied most extensively in patients with suspected appendicitis. These studies have found a relatively low sensitivity and a high false-positive rate for this test. The most useful aspect of CRP is its negative predictive value. Patients with abdominal pain for more than 12 hours and a normal CRP value have a very low probability (<2%) of acute appendicitis. To date, the usefulness of CRP determination in the evaluation of acute abdominal pain is unclear. Further investigation is needed before it can be recommended for routine use.

CERVICAL GRAM'S STAIN

A Gram's stain and culture of any cervical discharge is an important component of a complete pelvic examination in a woman presenting with acute abdominal pain. The swab should remain in the cervical os until thorough absorption occurs so that the smear is representative of the discharge. A clean slide should be lightly smeared with the discharge and dried before staining.

The most frequent finding on Gram's stain in patients with pelvic inflammatory disease (PID) is an increased number of polymorphonuclear leukocytes (>30 WBCs/HPF). The Gram's stain is most helpful in patients with gonococcal salpingitis: intracellular gram-negative diplococci are present in approximately two thirds of these patients. Unfortunately findings on Gram's stain are neither specific nor sensitive in many instances of endometritis and salpingitis, because specific bacteria may not be seen or the bacteria identified may not represent the actual causative organisms. An increasing number of pelvic infections are caused by chlamydia, mycoplasmas, and anaerobic bacterial species. These anaerobes include *Streptococcus*, *Bacteroides* and *Clostridium* species and are usually present along with aerobic bacteria. These nongonococcal organisms are best identified by growth on culture. In light of the complex microbiologic aspects of PID, the cervical Gram's stain can be a simple and potentially informative diagnostic test, but it is not reliable to predict the organisms involved in the infection.

RADIOGRAPHIC EVALUATION

The radiographic evaluation of a patient with acute abdominal pain can be helpful, particularly when radiographs reveal confirmatory information. Whereas abnormal findings on a radiograph are clearly informative, normal or inconclusive radiographs do not exclude a diagnosis and should be repeated if the clinical situation remains unresolved. Radiographs are not always needed, particularly when they will add nothing to an already clear clinical situation or when they may delay care in a critically ill patient. One should beware of radiographs of suboptimal quality, in which the techniques used are not adequate to demonstrate subtle findings.

Chest Radiographs
Posteroanterior and lateral chest radiographs obtained in the upright position should always be part of the diagnostic evaluation of a patient believed to have an intra-abdominal infection. These radiographs are particularly important in children and elderly patients, in whom pneumonia or other conditions confined to the thorax may account for acute abdominal symptoms. The characteristic radiologic findings of pneumonia may be absent early in the disease process, even when clinical findings are obvious. One should look for free intraperitoneal air, which is best seen between the apex of the diaphragm and the liver on the right side. An upright chest radiograph can detect as little as 1 cc of free intraperitoneal air. Upper GI disasters, such as gastric volvulus or Boerhaave's syndrome, may present with abnormal findings evident only on a chest radiograph.

Whenever a pleural effusion is noted on a chest radiograph, decubitus studies should be obtained. The involved hemithorax should be dependent. These radiographs provide a reasonable estimate of the presence and size of a pleural effusion and can demonstrate pulmonary consolidation, which may be obscured by an effusion on the upright radiograph.

Abdominal Radiographs
Radiographs of the abdomen in the supine and upright positions are essential to evaluate any patient with moderate to severe abdominal pain and tenderness when the decision for treatment cannot be made on the basis of clinical findings. A left lateral decubitus radiograph is a ready substitute for an

upright radiograph when the patient cannot stand. Positioning the patient upright or on the left side for 5 minutes before x-ray exposure is sufficient to detect small volumes of free intraperitoneal air.

A number of characteristics should be noted in studying abdominal radiographs. They include free intraperitoneal air, localized air, distribution of gas within the intestinal lumen, and demonstration of opacities.

Free Intraperitoneal Air. Free intraperitoneal air is seen best on upright or decubitus views between the opaque shadows of the liver and the diaphragm or body wall. This gas should be located at the apex of the diaphragm, which is the most superior portion on an upright radiograph. Failure to see free air at this location or failure to note a shift in location with a change in the position of the patient can lead to misinterpretation. The presence of free gas may represent perforation of a hollow viscus, but this finding is not uniformly present in patients with perforation of the GI tract. Detectable free intraperitoneal air is found most commonly in patients with a perforated gastric or duodenal ulcer; it is present in 80% of patients with these conditions.

Free intraperitoneal gas is commonly noted when abdominal radiographs are obtained during the first 2 weeks after celiotomy. Absorption of retained air after the operation may be slow, but the volume of air should decrease with time. There should never be an increase in the volume of air after an operation: this indicates perforation of a hollow viscus or an abscess.

Localized Air. Sites of air localized in the abdomen also can represent perforation of a viscus. Air from a duodenal perforation can outline the second portion of the duodenum or the right kidney. An intra-abdominal abscess may appear as multiple, localized, small gas bubbles. The presence of air in the biliary tree (pneumobilia) suggests a fistula between the biliary system and the intestine; it is always pathologic in the absence of a previous biliary-enteric bypass. Pylephlebitis, or air in the portal venous system, is an ominous finding; it usually occurs in association with severe intestinal ischemia.

Air within the intestinal wall (pneumatosis) is distinctly abnormal but must be taken in context with the findings of the physical examination. Although it may be associated with invasion of the intestinal wall by bacteria resulting from ischemia or mucosal destruction, pneumatosis also can be seen in patients with asymptomatic chronic obstructive pulmonary disease.

The presence of air within the wall of the gallbladder (emphysematous cholecystitis) is usually due to infection by *Clostridium perfringens,* but rarely it can occur from infection with other gas-forming bacteria.

Distribution of Gas Within the Intestinal Lumen. The appearance of more than a few areas of gas within the small intestine is distinctly abnormal. Alteration of the gas pattern within the intestinal lumen represents the key to the diagnosis of mechanical intestinal obstruction. Gas is normally found in the large intestine; however, when there is more proximal obstruction, colonic gas is

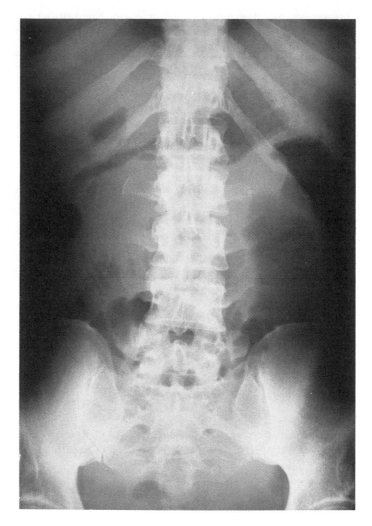

A

Figure 24. Small-intestinal obstruction. These flat (**A**) and upright (**B**) abdominal radiographs demonstrate distended loops of small intestine with air–fluid interfaces at varying heights in the same loop of intestine. No gas is identifiable within the colon.

passed and no longer appears on the radiograph. The findings of intestinal obstruction are much more evident as time passes. Thus, abdominal radiographs may not portray the classic findings of mechanical obstruction during the first 6 hours after the onset of symptoms. When there is doubt, the radiographs should be repeated.

Three key features of mechanical small-intestinal obstruction are evident on plain and upright radiographs: (1) the presence of distended hoop-shaped

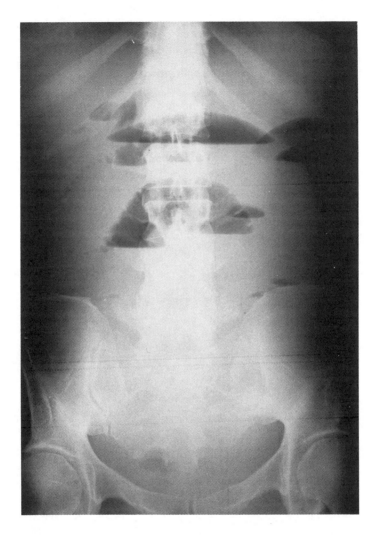

B

loops above the site of obstruction; (2) air–fluid levels within the intestinal lumen, particularly levels at different heights, which appear as an inverted J; and (3) the absence of gas in the colon (Fig. 24). Except in newborn infants, the small and large intestine can usually be differentiated. Plica circulares are prominent transverse markings that identify the small intestine and extend across the full diameter of the intestine. In contrast, haustral markings noted in colonic distention are limited to a portion of the diameter of the intestine.

Patients with high jejunal obstruction typically demonstrate little or no small-intestinal gas on radiographs, because the intestinal contents proximal to the obstruction are regurgitated into the stomach. When the obstruction occurs more distally, enlarged intestinal loops are aligned in parallel, giving a typical stepladder appearance on the supine radiograph. These distended loops are usually oriented obliquely from the right lower to the left upper quadrant on the upright radiograph. The area of obstruction is always below the lowest fluid level noted in the upright position. In scrutinizing the abdominal radiographs in a patient with mechanical obstruction, one should always search the areas of the pelvis and groin, where a tapering gas pattern may indicate the site of an incarcerated hernia.

An obstructed segment of small intestine incarcerated within the abdomen (closed-loop obstruction) can vary in appearance (Fig. 25). A patient

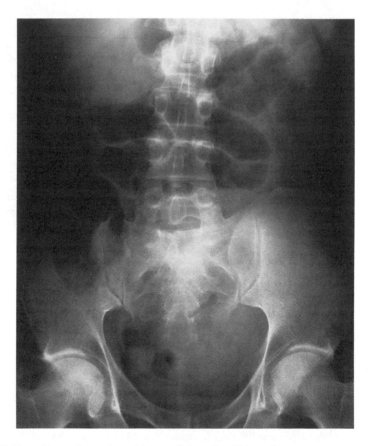

Figure 25. Closed-loop obstruction of the small intestine. This radio-graph shows laddering of segments of small intestine. There is no gas in the midabdomen.

with complete closed-loop obstruction has virtually no gas within the fluid-filled incarcerated segment, which may actually appear as a pseudotumor. When obstruction is incomplete, gas can accumulate in the incarcerated segment, producing a gas–fluid interface. The findings of a closed-loop obstruction can be easily overlooked; therefore, an absence of classic findings of intestinal obstruction on the plain abdominal radiographs should not lead to exclusion of this diagnosis.

In contrast to mechanical obstruction, paralytic ileus is accompanied by dilatation and intraluminal gas within segments of both the large and small intestines. The distribution of intraluminal gas in both the colon and the small intestine is a very important distinction between paralytic ileus and mechanical obstruction. With ileus, fluid accumulates in the intestine, and multiple air–fluid interfaces are present after a few hours. In contrast to mechanical obstruction, gas–fluid interfaces in paralytic ileus are usually at the same level in the segment of intestine, producing inverted U loops on the upright radiograph. Ogilvie's syndrome is a disorder in which paralytic ileus occurs predominantly in the colon; it can cause massive distention of the large intestine. Cecal distention can be progressive. A rapid change in the size of the colon or a cecal diameter of more than 12 cm is an important radiographic finding; it is associated with a high incidence of subsequent intestinal perforation or necrosis.

Mechanical colonic obstruction is less common than obstruction of the small intestine. Obstruction of the colon is usually due to a neoplasm or volvulus. The cecum is usually the most dilated portion of the colon, regardless of the point of obstruction (Fig. 26). When the outline of the gas-filled colon is followed across the abdomen, the point of obstruction can be identified by the abrupt disappearance of intraluminal gas in the colon.

Volvulus occurs in segments of the colon with a long and freely moveable mesentery, usually the sigmoid or cecum. The sigmoid colon is the most common site of volvulus, which is characterized by massive distention in which the convexity of the twisted sigmoid loop lies away from the point of obstruction (Fig. 26). Usually a midline mesenteric crease points toward the site of torsion in the pelvis. The radiographic features of colonic volvulus can be misinterpreted if this diagnosis is not considered.

Cecal volvulus is characterized by: (1) massive cecal distention with displacement of the cecum to the left upper quadrant; (2) a single air–fluid level within the cecum; (3) the aforementioned signs of small-intestinal obstruction; and (4) visualization of gas outlining the ileocecal valve on the right side of the cecum. Compromise of the cecal blood supply can lead to gangrene, but perforation occurs only when the ileocecal valve is competent and a closed-loop obstruction occurs.

Acute diverticulitis and intussusception can also cause colonic obstruction. Contrast enemas are often helpful to confirm the presence and to determine the site and cause of all colonic obstructions.

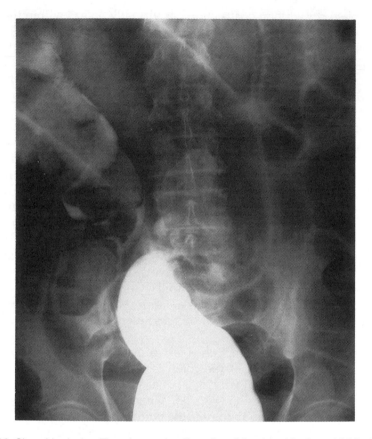

Figure 26. Sigmoid volvulus. There is massive distention of the sigmoid colon, which is displaced to the right upper abdomen. Contrast demonstrates the point of volvulus.

Patients with inflammatory bowel disease or *Clostridium difficile* entero-colitis can have toxic megacolon, which has the appearance on upright radiographs of distention of the transverse colon with a fluid level within this segment. In contrast to mechanical colonic obstruction, haustra may not be seen, and the transverse colon can assume a tubular appearance. Flat projections into the colonic lumen representing pseudopolyps can be evident on plain radiographs. There may be irregularities in the intestinal wall; these serrations represent ulcerations of the transverse colon. Characteristically, the hepatic and splenic flexures are situated in a normal position, and the length of the involved segments of intestine appear normal despite distention of the colon (Fig. 27).

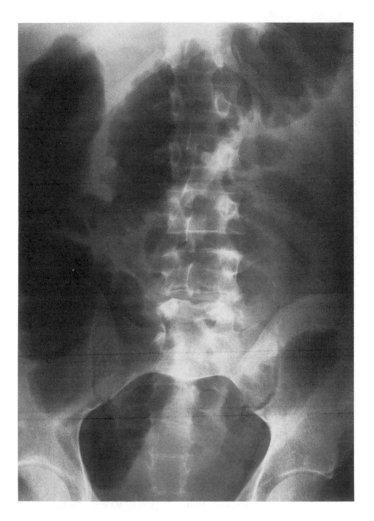

Figure 27. Toxic megacolon in a patient with ulcerative colitis. Serrations and ulcerative irregularities are visible in the transverse colon.

Demonstration of Opacities. Calcium-containing objects can be demonstrated on abdominal radiographs but are not always the cause of acute pain. Calculi can occur in the gallbladder (Fig. 28) and throughout the urinary tract. Pancreatic calcifications indicate the presence of chronic pancreatitis. Appendiceal fecaliths are seen in 25% of children younger than 2 years who have appendicitis. The incidence of fecaliths decreases with age; they are present in only 5% of adults. Phleboliths in the pelvis can be confused with ureteral cal-

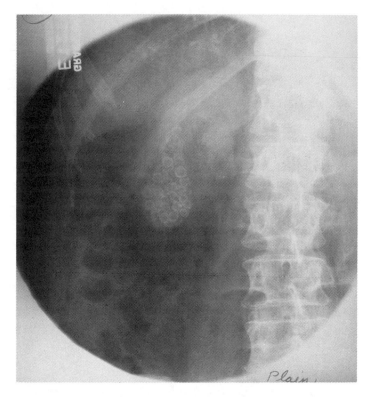

Figure 28. Upright abdominal radiograph demonstrating radiopaque gallstones. Only about 15% of gallstones will be visualized on plain radiographs of the abdomen.

culi; contrast studies of the urinary tract may be necessary to make this distinction.

Gallstone ileus is an infrequent cause of intestinal obstruction characterized by a visible calcified stone in the intestinal lumen, signs of small-intestinal obstruction, and pneumobilia or gas outlining the enterobiliary fistulous tract (Fig. 29). The terminal ileum is the most common site of obstruction because of its smaller diameter. When signs of colonic obstruction are present, the enterobiliary fistula usually communicates directly with the colon.

Thin, shell-like calcifications can outline the wall of an abdominal aortic aneurysm, but they also may be found with aneurysmal dilatation of other intra-abdominal vessels. A cross-table lateral radiograph is a sensitive indicator of calcification outlining an abdominal aortic aneurysm. The presence of eggshell calcifications more than 2 cm in diameter at other intra-abdominal sites indicates an arterial aneurysm that is at increased risk for rupture.

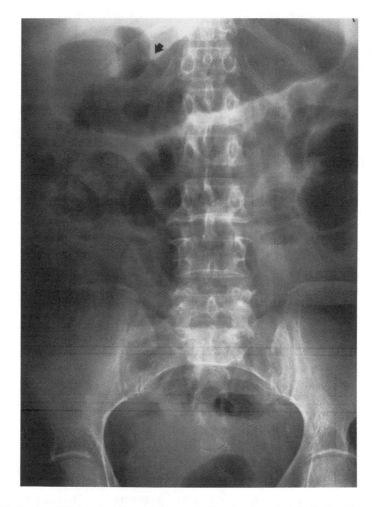

Figure 29. Supine abdominal radiograph demonstrating the characteristic findings in a gallstone ileus. The arrow identifies the fistulous tract outlined by air.

Other Findings. A number of subtle radiographic findings may add supportive evidence to the clinical diagnosis of acute abdominal pain, but they are nonspecific. In the absence of arthritic changes, scoliosis may be due to splinting of the psoas or paravertebral muscles when there is an inflammatory process involving the retroperitoneum. Inflammatory processes also can obliterate the preperitoneal flank stripe or psoas shadow on the side of the abnormality.

The presence of a large amount of intra-abdominal fluid gives a ground-glass appearance to the abdominal radiograph. The psoas shadows may be indistinct, and the preperitoneal flank stripes bulge outward. If the intestine is gas-filled, the excess fluid widens the space separating the loops of intestine. These signs do not distinguish whether the intra-abdominal fluid is due to hemorrhage, ascites, or peritonitis.

A space-occupying mass can displace loops of intestine or other viscera. The mass may be uniformly opaque and may represent an enlarged intra-abdominal organ. Although the radiographic density of an abscess may appear uniform, irregularities in density often are noted, particularly when gas-forming bacteria are present in the abscess. When a subphrenic abscess is present, radiographs may show elevation of the ipsilateral hemidiaphragm, and there is often an effusion in the adjacent pleural space.

Intravenous Nephropyelography

Emergency nephropyelography can assist in the diagnosis of abdominal pain caused by urinary tract obstruction, usually a result of ureteral calculi. With ureteral obstruction, there may be a delay in excretion of contrast medium by the kidney or mild dilatation of the collection system proximal to the point of obstruction. Delayed excretion accompanied by an identifiable calculus in the ureter establishes the diagnosis of a ureteral stone.

Emergency Barium Enema Study

A barium enema should never be performed when intestinal gangrene or perforation is suspected. When mechanical obstruction of the colon is suggested by plain abdominal radiographs, a barium enema may demonstrate the site and cause of obstruction. An emergency barium enema also can be helpful to make the diagnosis of intestinal obstruction in newborn infants. In children with intussusception, hydrostatic reduction of the intussusception by barium enema can be therapeutic.

An emergency barium enema study has been suggested as an adjunct for the diagnosis of acute appendicitis, particularly in patients who are at increased operative risk or may have other causes for their abdominal pain. This study is done without any intestinal preparation, and a 1-m hydrostatic column should be used to limit the pressure from infusion. The following criteria suggest acute appendicitis: (1) lack of filling of the appendix; (2) a mass effect indenting the medial or inferior cecal wall or terminal ileum; (3) mucosal irregularities of the terminal ileum; and (4) partial filling of the appendix with mucosal abnormalities within the appendiceal lumen (Fig. 30). One must remember that lack of filling of the appendix occurs in one tenth of the healthy population. These findings are subjective and can occur because of other sources of inflammation in the right lower quadrant. The diagnostic accuracy of this study improves when multiple abnormalities are identified. An emergency barium enema examination should be used selectively because the false-positive rate is about 10 percent.

Upper Gastrointestinal Radiographic Series

An upper GI radiographic series is rarely useful in a patient with acute abdominal pain. When the diagnosis is confusing, however, a contrast examination of the upper GI tract may demonstrate an unsuspected perforated ulcer. This study also may be helpful in instances of high small-intestinal obstruction when plain radiographs are normal. Water-soluble contrast material is preferred when perforation is suspected; otherwise barium should be used. In unusual instances, a contrast examination of the small intestine may help differentiate between mechanical obstruction and paralytic ileus, particularly when contrast medium readily passes into the colon. In the unusual instance of gastric volvulus, an upper GI contrast examination shows the abnormal rotation of the stomach and failure of contrast medium to pass the pylorus.

Ultrasonography

Abdominal ultrasonography can be useful in the diagnosis of acute abdominal diseases, but its specificity and sensitivity are operator-dependent. An ultrasonographic examination is best used to confirm a suspected clinical diagnosis of localized abdominal pain and to exclude other, less frequent causes of pain.

Ultrasonography can confirm the presence of gallstones in a patient believed to have acute cholecystitis with 85% to 90% accuracy; it is most accurate when the gallstones are larger than 3 mm in diameter. The following features must be present to diagnose stones in the gallbladder: (1) an echogenic focus within the gallbladder lumen; (2) gravitational movement of this focus with changes in position; and (3) the presence of an acoustic shadow immediately subjacent to echogenic focus. The demonstration of all three of these criteria is 100% predictive for the presence of gallstones.

Sonographic findings suggestive of acute cholecystitis include thickening of the gallbladder wall, focal abnormalities of the gallbladder wall, and pericholecystic fluid. On the basis of these criteria, ultrasonography can have a positive predictive value of more than 90% for acute cholecystitis. An ultrasonographic examination can accurately demonstrate enlargement of the common bile duct or intrahepatic duct, but most often it does not detect common bile duct stones. Early common bile duct obstruction can be present without demonstrable ductal dilatation. Ultrasonography also can exclude an abnormality of the liver or kidney as the cause of right upper quadrant pain.

Ultrasonography may be helpful to confirm the diagnosis of pancreatitis, particularly if gland edema, a pseudocyst, or a peripancreatic fluid collection is noted. In approximately 30% of examinations, the pancreatic head and distal common bile duct are hidden by overlying intestinal gas. Ultra-

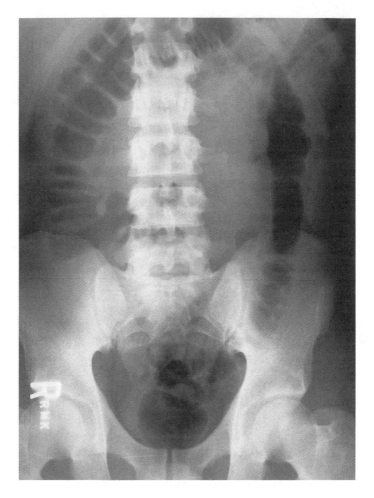

A

Figure 30. (**A**) Flat abdominal radiograph and (**B**) contrast enema study in a patient with acute appendicitis. There is a mass effect upon the cecum and no contrast in the appendix.

sonography can demonstrate an abdominal aortic aneurysm; it is very accurate in determining the size of the aneurysm.

Sonographic imaging has also been used in the diagnosis of acute appendicitis. The examination is performed with a high resolution transducer; it involves graded compression of the surrounding intestinal loops. Patient cooperation is mandatory, and intravenous analgesia is often required. The criteria for acute appendicitis are the demonstration of a noncompressible

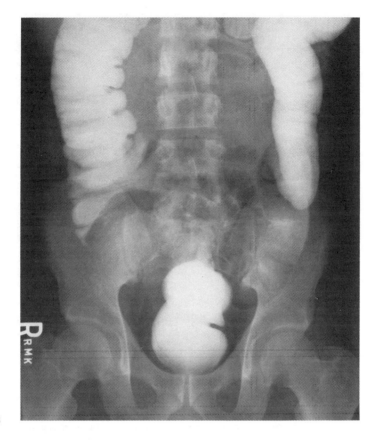

B

appendix that is greater than 7 mm in diameter (Fig. 31) or the presence of an appendicolith in a patient with symptoms. In most healthy patients, the appendix is not visible on ultrasonography. Reported sensitivity rates with this technique range from 75% to 95%. The findings on ultrasonography also can suggest an alternative diagnosis, such as mesenteric adenitis or gynecologic disease, in patients with acute right lower quadrant abdominal pain.

Ultrasonography is often the best initial imaging modality for women with acute pelvic pain. If the HCG test is positive, ultrasonography should be used to determine whether an intrauterine or an ectopic pregnancy is present. If the HCG test is negative, ultrasonography may demonstrate a hydrosalpinx, ovarian enlargement, a tubo-ovarian abscess, or an ovarian cyst.

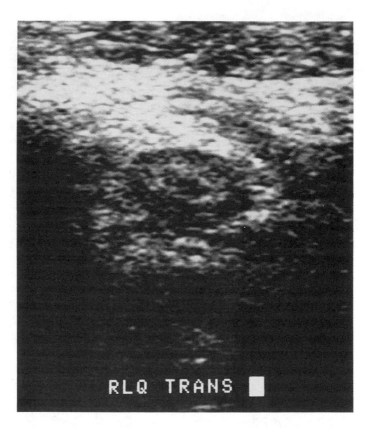

Figure 31. Ultrasound of the right lower quadrant in a patient with equivocal signs and symptoms of appendicitis. This transverse section displays a "target sign," which is the inflamed serosa and mucosa of the appendix. Longitudinal sections disclosed a sausage-shaped mass. Gross and microscopic pathologic findings were consistent with acute appendicitis.

Computed Tomography

Computed tomography (CT) of the abdomen can play an important role in the diagnosis of an acute abdomen. The optimal study requires the use of both intravenous and oral contrast media. Intra-abdominal structures are visualized in detail without being hidden by intestinal gas. Therefore CT is often the preferred study for imaging the pancreas and other retroperitoneal structures. Free intraperitoneal air, pneumobilia, and intraperitoneal fluid are readily visible on CT. Retroperitoneal or extramural gas suggesting an abscess or intestinal ischemia can also be visualized, making CT the most accurate examination for detection of an intra-abdominal abscess.

Findings on CT that suggest an acute inflammatory process include thickening of the intestinal wall, obliteration of normal fat planes, mesenteric edema, fascial thickening, and abnormal fluid collections. These findings can indicate the presence of acute diseases such as pancreatitis, appendicitis, or diverticulitis. CT is often indicated in patients with suspected acute diverticulitis but without signs of generalized peritonitis, both to confirm the diagnosis and to exclude complications such as an associated abscess.

Other conditions that can cause acute abdominal pain and can be detected by CT include splenic infarction, acute cholecystitis, intussusception, Crohn's disease, abdominal wall or retroperitoneal hemorrhage, incarcerated hernia, aortic dissection or rupture, urinary tract lithiasis, nephritis, and traumatic injury to the intra-abdominal organs. Finally, CT-guided aspiration of abdominal fluid collections may be indicated in selected patients for diagnostic or therapeutic reasons.

Angiography

When clinical findings suggest intestinal ischemia and physical signs of peritonitis are absent, arteriography of the mesenteric vessels is indicated. Superior mesenteric angiography can distinguish arterial from venous occlusion and also can help distinguish low cardiac output syndromes from embolic events. Some authors have reported improved results in the treatment of nonembolic small-intestinal ischemia by infusion of vasodilating agents directly into the superior mesenteric vessels.

Radionuclide Scanning

Radionuclide scanning with various technetium-labeled iminodiacetic acids (IDA) has been useful for the diagnosis of acute cholecystitis. This test does not require intestinal absorption and is not influenced by intestinal gas, body habitus, or mild abnormalities of liver function. Scans with IDA have an overall accuracy of more than 90%, but they are less accurate if the serum bilirubin level exceeds 10 mg/100mL.

This test requires uptake of the radionuclide by hepatocytes and its excretion into the biliary tract. After the labeled IDA compound is given, scans are taken every 5 minutes for the first 30 minutes and then at longer intervals. If the gallbladder is not visualized within 1 hour, delayed scans should be done at intervals of up to 4 hours.

Demonstration of radionuclide within the gallbladder within 1 hour indicates cystic duct patency; acute cholecystitis is highly unlikely in this setting. Lack of filling of the gallbladder or delayed visualization may represent either acute or chronic obstruction of the cystic duct. The appearance of radionuclide in the gallbladder 1 to 4 hours after it is administered usually indicates the presence of chronic gallbladder disease, but there can be some overlap between acute and chronic cholecystitis when delayed visualization occurs. If no radionuclide activity appears in the intestine within 4 hours de-

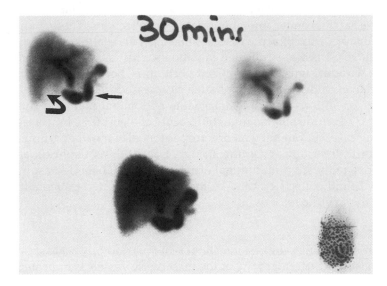

Figure 32. HIDA scan of a patient with right upper quadrant abdominal pain. Radionuclide is seen within the lumen of the bowel at 30 minutes (arrow). The area of the gallbladder (curved arrow) failed to accumulate any radionuclide even after 2 hours. Gross and microscopic findings were consistent with acute cholecystitis.

spite prompt uptake by the hepatocytes, common bile duct obstruction is present (Fig. 32).

CULDOCENTESIS

Culdocentesis is occasionally useful in selected patients with PID or believed to have a ruptured ectopic pregnancy, although use of this procedure has become limited with advances in laparoscopic techniques and ultrasonography. Contraindications to culdocentesis include a retroflexed uterus and the presence of a solid mass within the cul-de-sac. More than 5 WBCs/HPF of aspirate indicate PID or another inflammatory process in the pelvis, such as perforative appendicitis. In patients with PID, culdocentesis can provide material for culture and Gram's stain, which may be particularly useful in recurrent infections or those not responding to standard treatment. Many instances of PID are not associated with large amounts of pus in the cul-de-sac.

The return of nonclotting blood on culdocentesis indicates a ruptured ectopic pregnancy, ruptured corpus luteum cyst, or other source of hemoperitoneum. Because most ectopic pregnancies are diagnosed with a combination of the β-HCG test, transabdominal or transvaginal ultrasonography, and laparoscopy, culdocentesis is usually unnecessary.

ELECTROCARDIOGRAM

An electrocardiogram is usually not helpful in the diagnosis of acute abdominal pain. The presence of acute myocardial infarction or atrial fibrillation, however, may indicate that the pain is related to intestinal ischemia caused by low cardiac output or an embolus arising from the heart. A normal electrocardiogram does not necessarily exclude myocardial infarction as a cause for abdominal pain.

DIAGNOSTIC PARACENTESIS

Diagnostic paracentesis—a peritoneal tap—is useful to establish the diagnosis of primary peritonitis in patients with cirrhosis or chronic renal failure. Primary peritonitis is suggested when a peritoneal tap reveals more than 300 WBCs/mL with a differential count exhibiting more than 30% granulocytes. Confirmatory clinical findings and growth of bacteria on culture are necessary because on routine sampling about 30% of patients with cirrhosis with noninfected ascites also have a peritoneal WBC count in this range.

Abdominal paracentesis and peritoneal lavage also have been used in the diagnosis of nontraumatic acute abdominal pain or secondary bacterial peritonitis. A paracentesis that returns brown or malodorous fluid, bile, or fluid with demonstrable bacteria on Gram's stain represents secondary bacterial peritonitis. These diagnostic studies always should be performed after a radiographic examination because about 25% of diagnostic taps cause a pneumoperitoneum detectable on a radiograph.

The reported accuracy of diagnostic peritoneal lavage for evaluation of abdominal pain ranges from 60% to 95%. Diagnostic lavage is performed by inserting a peritoneal dialysis catheter into the peritoneum, usually under direct vision. One liter of normal saline solution is infused into the peritoneal cavity, and the effluent is returned by the siphoning effect of gravity drainage. More than 10^5 RBCs/mL or 500 WBCs/mL of effluent is considered a positive test. False-negative results are unusual, but they can occur in patients with acute biliary disease or those with localized peritonitis or an intraabdominal abscess. False-positive results can occur in patients with mesenteric adenitis, acute diverticulitis, acute pancreatitis, and PID. This study is most useful for patients believed to have peritonitis but whose physical findings are equivocal or unreliable and for whom other studies cannot be performed or are not diagnostic.

LAPAROSCOPY

Laparoscopy is an invasive diagnostic study that allows for direct visualization of the intraperitoneal contents. Advances in equipment and video technology, along with the advent of laparoscopic cholecystectomy, have led to a renewed interest among surgeons in the applications of diagnostic laparoscopy. Laparoscopy is a relatively safe procedure, although there is a small risk of visceral injury, wound infection, and potential adverse hemodynamic effects of pneumoperitoneum from insufflation of carbon dioxide. Although diagnostic laparoscopy can be performed with local anesthesia, general anesthesia is more commonly used for evaluation of an acute abdomen.

Laparoscopy can be an important diagnostic tool when an exact diagnosis of acute abdominal pain cannot be made by clinical assessment, laboratory tests, or radiographic studies. Several recent reports have shown that the selective use of diagnostic laparoscopy can improve the overall accuracy in the evaluation of an acute abdomen. They can also lower the rates of unnecessary laparotomy while decreasing the incidence of delay in diagnosis or treatment.

Laparoscopy may be particularly beneficial in several clinical situations. Historically, the reported rate of misdiagnosis in patients with possible appendicitis has ranged from 10% to 20% overall, and the negative appendectomy rate can be as high as 40% in women of child-bearing age. A normal appendix can be identified at laparoscopy more than 90% of the time, and failure to see a normal appendix suggests appendicitis is present. Gynecologic disorders that may cause acute abdominal pain, including PID, ovarian cyst, tubo-ovarian abscess, endometriosis, and ectopic pregnancy, often can be demonstrated. Laparoscopy also can have a therapeutic role when an inflamed appendix is identified, because laparoscopic appendectomy can be done safely in many patients. Other unusual causes of abdominal pain such as tuberculous peritonitis can be confirmed by laparoscopy and peritoneal biopsy.

Evaluation of abdominal pain in elderly patients often can be difficult because of factors such as an inadequately given history, disordered mental status, alteration in physical findings, and nonspecific laboratory or radiologic examinations. The clinical diagnosis of mesenteric ischemia is notoriously difficult to establish in a timely way because the physical signs and radiographic findings often are subtle and nonspecific. Laparoscopy allows direct visualization of the intestine and may improve the rapidity and accuracy of diagnosis in this group of patients. Laparoscopy can be a valuable diagnostic tool in patients who have unreliable physical examinations, including immunocompromised patients, patients receiving steroids, those in intensive care units for conditions unrelated to the abdomen, and patients with spinal cord injuries.

Because of its invasive nature, potential complications, and relative expense, a selective approach to the use of laparoscopy is reasonable. This procedure should be considered, however, in patients with acute abdominal pain when the need for operative intervention is indeterminate on the basis of clinical and radiographic evaluation.

SUGGESTED READING

Carroll BA. Preferred imaging techniques for the diagnosis of cholecystitis and cholelithiasis. *Ann Surg.* 1989; 210:1.

Dueholm S, Bagi P, Bud M. Laboratory aid in the diagnosis of acute appendicitis. *Dis Colon Rectum.* 1989; 32:855–859.

Eisenberg RL, Heineken P, Hedgcock MW, et al. Evaluation of plain abdominal radiographs in the diagnosis of abdominal pain. *Ann Intern Med.* 1982; 97:257.

Laing FC. Ultrasonography of the acute abdomen. *Radiol Clin North Am.* 1992; 30:389–404.

Ogilvie H. Large intestine colic due to sympathetic deprivation: a new clinical syndrome. *Br Med J.* 1948; 2:671.

Patterson-Brown S. The acute abdomen: the role of laparoscopy. *Ballieres Clin Gastroenterol.* 1991; 5:691–703.

Plewa MC. Emergency abdominal radiography. *Emerg Med Clin North Am.* 1991; 9:827–852.

Prego L, Gronner AT, Glazer M, et al. Imaging of the nontraumatic acute abdomen. *Emerg Med Clin North Am.* 1989; 7:453–496.

Richardson JD, Flint LM, Polk HC Jr. Peritoneal lavage: a useful diagnostic adjuvant for peritonitis. *Surgery.* 1983; 94:826–829.

Shaff MI, Tarr RW, Partain CL, et al. Computed tomography and magnetic resonance imaging of the acute abdomen. *Surg Clin North Am.* 1988; 68:233–254.

CHAPTER 5

■

Appendicitis

Joseph M. Vitello, MD

The most important clinical problem afflicting the vermiform appendix is acute inflammation. Appendicitis is one of the most common acute surgical diseases of the abdomen. It affects approximately 6% of the population. The peak incidence of the disease is the second and third decades of life. A fecalith obstructing the lumen remains the prevalent, albeit not the solitary, pathophysiologic mechanism of the condition. One of the clinician's goals is to diagnose and treat appendicitis before the disease progresses to perforation and peritonitis. The other goal is to avoid an unnecessary operation on patients who do not have a condition that requires surgical intervention. Because perforation leads to morbidity and occasionally death, the clinical goal is an early diagnosis.

In most instances the diagnosis of appendicitis is straightforward and readily confirmed by procurement of a compatible history, a consistent physical examination, and a few corroborative laboratory tests. Despite technologic advances and a plethora of available sophisticated tests, appendicitis remains a *clinical* diagnosis. It is a gratifying clinical experience when the history and physical examination alone lead to the correct diagnosis and surgical removal of the diseased organ results in recovery of the patient.

The diagnosis of appendicitis, however, may be obscure and problematic, especially in very young or very old patients. Fortunately, the disorder is uncommon at the extremes of life. With appendicitis it is typical to have an atypical picture. As Charles McBurney wrote, "One cannot with accuracy determine from the symptoms the extent and severity of the disease." Even superb clinicians occasionally have difficulty detecting acute appendicitis. Patients may have few symptoms, even when they have gangrenous or perforative appendicitis. Conversely, a patient may exhibit signs of diffuse peritonitis but may have only early, localized appendicitis. These diverse, atypical signs and symptoms may cause confusion. They accentuate the need to master the nuances of disease detection.

The diagnosis of acute appendicitis has three components: a history compatible with appendicitis; a reliable physical examination; and laboratory findings that support the physical findings. Any two of the three components reasonably secure the diagnosis or at least justify surgical intervention.

THE PATIENT HISTORY

The classic history and physical findings of nonperforating appendicitis follow a reasonably consistent pattern. They progress in the following manner: (1) anorexia; (2) mild to moderate, poorly localized midabdominal pain; (3) nausea and vomiting; (4) pain migrating to the right lower quadrant (RLQ); (5) localized tenderness or guarding over the appendix; (6) muscular rigidity or "peritoneal signs" in the RLQ; (7) fever and leukocytosis, which may or may not occur. The events typically occur in this order in acute appendicitis.

Knowledge of the pathophysiology of appendicitis aids in understanding the signs and symptoms of acute appendicitis. After a fecalith occludes the lumen, the appendix distends because of continued secretion of mucus. Stimulation of the visceral afferent pain fibers produces a dull, poorly localized, diffuse or midabdominal pain. Peristalsis may be stimulated so early in the course of the disease that the pain may be paroxysmal. As the distention worsens, so does the intensity of the visceral pain, causing a constant, boring discomfort. Ultimately the inflammation involves the serosa of the appendix and the parietal peritoneal surface. At this juncture, tenderness localizes at McBurney's point. (McBurney described tenderness to the pressure of one finger, regardless of where the appendix lay, exactly $1\frac{1}{2}$ to 2 inches from the anterior superior iliac spine on a straight line drawn from that structure to the umbilicus. This point corresponds to the point at which the appendix attaches to the cecum.) Therefore the sensation shifts from a poorly localized discomfort to a constant, moderately intense, precisely defined pain. As the inflammatory reaction progresses, peritoneal irritation becomes increasingly evident and is accompanied by a rising fever and leukocytosis. If the disease remains undiagnosed, perforation occurs. The pain may abate temporarily on perforation because the obstructing fecalith is relieved, but this situation is uncommon.

To begin taking the patient's history, the physician should place him- or herself in a chair at the patient's bedside in such a way as to hold a conversation with the patient. Too often the physician rushes through this important aspect of disease detection. It is necessary to dissect carefully the sequence of events in search of subtle details.

Appetite

Anorexia has been stated by many authors to be essential in the diagnosis of appendicitis. This is probably an overstatement. What is true is that maintenance of a normal appetite with evolving appendicitis is uncommon. Loss of appetite *preceding* the development of abdominal pain is a reliable first finding. It should be specifically sought in the history because patients do not routinely note or offer this association spontaneously. It is worthwhile to ask when the patient last ate and if the amount consumed is considered normal intake. Diminution of the usual appetite may be a subtle finding. Most patients with appendicitis do note some degree of anorexia if asked about it. However, if the inflammatory process is contained by the omentum or in the retroperitoneal space, the initial anorexia may be nonexistent or trivial. Some patients with acute appendicitis temporarily improve with hospitalization, bed rest, and hydration. Their appetite returns, yet appendicitis may still exist. Therefore, reversal of the anorexia is not a reliable sign in excluding the diagnosis of acute appendicitis. Failure to appreciate this fact may delay intervention.

Pain

Abdominal pain is the chief symptom of acute appendicitis and typically *follows* the anorexia. It is worth spending a few minutes detailing the nature and characteristics of the onset of the pain. The patient often ascribes the pain to something he or she ate. As a rule, the discomfort does not develop rapidly but slowly progresses as a diffuse, intermittent, or constant pain in the epigastrium or around the umbilicus. This is an important detail in the history. The pain is distinctly unlike that of a perforated ulcer or ruptured ovarian cyst, in which the symptoms tend to be hyperacute and severe from the start. When the pain begins suddenly in the RLQ and is severe, with signs of rebound pain at the onset, it is unlikely that appendicitis is the cause. Appendicitis, however, can be a great fooler, and uncommonly the pain *is* very intense from the beginning. It starts in the RLQ, and the patient is writhing.

Often, the findings may be minimal in the early phase of the disease. The laboratory findings are usually normal. The physician may question the reliability of the patient or suspect a nonsurgical cause of the problem and send the patients home. A previously healthy patient's abdominal pain should not be attributed to neurosis. Healthy people who make the effort to travel to the emergency department in the middle of the night complaining of vague abdominal pain probably should be admitted to the hospital and appendicitis considered in the differential diagnosis of their complaint. The average person may experience a variety of abdominal pains throughout the course of time but does not rush to an emergency department with each episode. Though a patient does not know the diagnosis, the pain of a major abdominal illness is typically different enough to cause the patient to seek medical attention. Pain that awakens someone from a sound sleep is generally pathologic and not psychosomatic and should always be considered real.

Classically, the initial pain is centered over the midabdomen or lower epigastrium. Some authors state that the early pain of appendicitis is periumbilical, connoting that the pain is in or around the umbilicus. A point of clarification is in order. The visceral pain of early appendicitis is poorly localized but is perceived to be midabdomen. This is not referred pain. Actually, the pain tends to be diffuse or radiate out from a central, umbilical location, like the spokes of a wheel. The patient frequently passes an open hand over the midabdomen to delineate the location of the pain. The pain is episodic or occasionally constant. It may be mild or moderately severe in quality. Over a variable period of time (as little as 4 to 6 hours or as long as 24 to 48 hours) the aching migrates to the RLQ and remains there. Pain migration and localization are not pathognomonic for appendicitis, but they are common and are valuable signs when present. After the pain migrates, a dull, constant, severe discomfort usually settles in the RLQ. By this point in the disease most patients have a real sense of illness. If at work, many now seek medical attention or wish to leave for the day. Occasionally, there is no radiation of the pain and it starts in the RLQ. In this situation local irritation producing pain at the site of the appendix may be the only symptom. Why the pain is only perceived as starting in the RLQ in some circumstances is unclear.

The pain at this migratory juncture tends to be more severe than the initial vague central ache. However, it can be subtle enough that a variety of maneuvers will become necessary to elicit this pain. Knowledge of the most common anatomic positions of the appendix will lead to recognition in alterations of pain patterns and location. With a retrocecal appendix, for example, there may be a predominance of back or flank pain and a paucity of anterior abdominal complaints. A long retrocecal appendix can present with right upper quadrant pain and give the illusion of cholecystitis. Recently, however, some authors have refuted this and believe the retrocecal location does not alter the time to presentation, overall physical findings, or laboratory results. Variability in a pelvic location may lead to complaints of pain in the inguinal or suprapubic area or even left-sided abdominal pain. As mentioned, this pain pattern occurs over the course of several hours or 2 to 3 days. In acute appendicitis, symptoms beyond this are the symptoms of perforation. Patients with symptoms for many days or weeks probably do not have acute appendicitis.

Nausea and Vomiting

Distention and obstruction of any luminal structure will produce nausea and vomiting. These two symptoms occur early with appendicitis and tend to be at the onset of the anorexia or soon thereafter. Vomiting is said to occur in about 75% of patients with acute appendicitis but typically is not protracted. Many patients become nauseated at the thought of food. Typically, I inquire as to whether a favorite food would sound appealing. If appendicitis exists, most patients decline their favorite meal or experience nausea at the mere thought. Nausea and vomiting are thought to occur less commonly with retrocecal and retroileal appendicitis. Vomiting may be more prominent in children.

Tenderness and Guarding

The historical report of pain with coughing or with the bumpy car ride to the hospital suggest RLQ peritoneal irritation and should be sought in the history. Characteristically, by this stage of peritoneal inflammation, patients with acute appendicitis prefer not to move. They will splint or hold their side when coughing. They will walk with a slight lean toward the right in an attempt to protect their RLQ from unnecessary movement. This behavior may be observed during the patient interview and is invaluable.

Other Signs and Symptoms

As appendicitis progresses, an ileus may develop, leading to constipation or at least decreased frequency of the normal bowel habit. Diarrhea, in contradistinction, is not a common component of acute appendicitis, except possibly in the patient with missed appendicitis (smoldering, walled off, retrocecal abscess). These patients may present with diarrhea, especially if the abscess is lying over the rectosigmoid colon. Because diarrhea is less common, it tends to mislead the examiner when it does occur. Watery, loose stools early on in the history are very atypical and should raise concern about the validity of the diagnosis. Diarrhea may be more common in children than in older patients.

When deviation from this typical history is found, it is usually in a stoic individual who fails to heed natural warning signs. A contained perforation may then occur, with details of the antecedent illness obscure. Typically, this patient may have been going about his or her normal daily activities with only a minor ache, until fever, chills, or persistent pain demanded medical attention. Once there is diffuse peritonitis, the diagnosis of acute appendicitis is more difficult, because any of a number of conditions could lead to that end. However, with a thorough historical account of the events leading up to the peritonitis, the diagnosis often can still be gleaned.

Intestinal nonrotation, either partial or complete, can be responsible for an occasional puzzling pain pattern because of the unanticipated location of the appendix. This situation, while rare, should be remembered.

THE PHYSICAL EXAMINATION

A thorough physical examination should always be performed, despite the patient's only complaint of abdominal pain, since many disease entities present with abdominal pain but are nonsurgical. If a reliable history has been obtained, a clear concept of the patient's complaints can guide the examination. Physical findings will depend on the: (1) reliability of the patient, (2) timing of the presentation, and (3) location of the appendix. When there is confusion regarding the diagnosis, it is not unreasonable to admit the patient to the hospital for active observation whereby repeated abdominal examinations may be conveniently performed, preferably by the same examiner to minimize subjective findings. In this way, evolving signs such as pain migration or localization or objective improvement facilitates an accurate diagnosis.

The administration of pain medication before evaluation of a tender abdomen deserves comment. Classically, it is considered taboo to administer narcotics to a patient with abdominal pain prior to a definitive diagnosis. The rationale is that it may mask important physical findings, such as subtle rebound. This is generally true. However, an occasional adult or child patient will be apprehensive or have an exaggerated pain response, making a reliable examination impossible. An experienced examiner can judiciously medicate such an individual and find the physical examination is facilitated and more meaningful. I would advise a small intravenous dose of a pure narcotic agonist (1 to 4 mg morphine). This can always be reversed with naloxone, if necessary.

Vital Signs

Begin the physical examination by obtaining the vital signs. A normal temperature is common with early appendicitis, especially at the stages of anorexia, vague pain, and vomiting. The temperature, if elevated is usually only 99° to 100° F. As the disease progresses to RLQ rebound tenderness, a temperature of 101° F is not uncommon but not mandatory either. Fever in excess of 102° F is usually, but not always, associated with perforated appendicitis. A febrile state above 102° F very early in the disease process (history less than 8 hours) and without associated peritonitis, is unusual and should suggest an alternative cause of the symptoms. Fever does not always correlate with the severity of the inflammation. Gangrenous appendicitis may develop with or without fever. Some unusual instances of appendicitis begin with chills and high fever, but this is infrequent.

The pulse rate is usually normal in uncomplicated acute appendicitis and therefore not of much diagnostic aid. Tachycardia, when present, is due to dehydration and high fever and suggests perforation and peritonitis. Even in suppurative appendicitis, the pulse will be normal unless the patient is dehydrated and azotemic or has developed a high fever.

The physical examination of the abdomen should start with inspection, be followed by auscultation and percussion, and culminate with palpation. A comfortable room and adequate covering will ensure that the patient does not shiver or tense the abdominal wall because of the environmental conditions or embarrassment.

Inspection

Look at the patient. The eyes are basic to your assessment skills. Avoid the obsessive compulsion that many examiners possess to rush in and palpate the abdomen. Much useful information is gleaned by observing a patient's facial expression before, during, and after palpation of the abdomen or during changes in patient position. The patient who looks well, smiles or laughs with palpation of the RLQ, probably does not have appendicitis. If the patient coughs vigorously and holds his or her RLQ (Dunphy's sign) or refuses to cough because of pain, RLQ peritonitis is confirmed. This can be a sign of subtle, localized peritonitis without the physician's even placing a hand upon the patient! Additional maneuvers include asking the patient to arise from bed. The patient who jumps up easily and vigorously has no localizing signs. Individuals with evolving appendicitis will get up gingerly, splinting or holding the right side. If asked to walk across the room, a patient with appendicitis will ambulate gingerly and with a rightward-bent gait to avoid the exacerbation of RLQ pain. Finally, asking the patient to hop up and down on the right foot will exaggerate the pain of evolving appendicitis.

Next, look at the abdomen and the position the patient assumes. Are there any scars? Could the patient have had an incidental appendectomy without being aware of it? Patients with retrocecal appendicitis may lie supine, with the right leg flexed to keep the inflammatory mass of the appendix from lying on the psoas muscle (a visual psoas sign). With a proper history and this finding alone, the diagnosis is almost assured.

Auscultation

Next, warm up the stethoscope and auscultate the bowel sounds. Many patients, especially children, will develop voluntary guarding immediately if the stethoscope is cold. In early appendicitis, the bowel sounds are relatively normal and maintained or only mildly hypoactive. In perforated appendicitis with diffuse peritonitis, bowel sounds become absent. In between, a full spectrum develops. One thing is typical: the bowel sounds are usually *not* hyperactive, as may occur in the abdominal pain of gastroenteritis or intestinal obstruction. In addition, the stethoscope can be used to distract the wary or uncooperative patient. Attention is diverted by an individual listening to the patient's abdomen for the course of a minute or two. The patient does not suspect that the examiner has any alternative motive but to listen, yet slight downward pressure with the stethoscope on the abdominal wall while auscultating can be a method of indirect palpation. The distracted patient who is malingering often will not complain of pain, yet when directly palpated with the hand complains bitterly and excessively. This technique is also helpful in the uncooperative child.

Percussion

Percussion of the abdomen is an elegant way to detect peritoneal irritation without causing undue discomfort to the patient. The point of maximal tenderness can sometimes be located by this technique alone. Percussion should start at a point furthest from the patient's perceived tenderness. With advanced parietal inflammation, percussion in the left lower quadrant will produce RLQ rebound tenderness. This is a subtle Rovsing's sign. An experienced examiner can detect peritonitis without even placing a hand upon the abdomen by accidentally hitting the bed as the examiner approaches for the interview. Being shaken at the hips is akin to a bumpy car ride and allows the examiner to note sites of maximal tenderness. Directly percussing over McBurney's point is a more skillful way to test for early rebound pain, rather than pressing deeply and suddenly letting go. This latter method will frequently elicit "rebound tenderness" in many patients, especially children, even when parietal inflammation is not a component of the illness. This often leads to the overdiagnosis of peritonitis.

Palpation

Next begin a gentle palpation of the abdomen. Warm the examining hands, since patients may voluntarily guard from a cold hand. Start at a point furthest from the pain. If the most tender area is explored first, the patient becomes uncooperative and fearful of pain. The subsequent attempt at palpation may then be ruined, since the patient will display voluntary guarding. This is particularly true in children. Once a methodical, gentle palpation searching for tenderness is completed, the process should be repeated with a slightly more aggressive examining hand. Attempt now to detect not only more deep-seated tenderness but also any mass. The examiner should really *feel* the abdomen. Too often the examination is cursorily and hastily performed without attention to the exact location of discomfort. Palpate both sides of the abdomen simultaneously, with both hands; that is, palpate the left side of the abdomen with your right hand and the right side of the abdomen with your left hand. This is the best way to detect voluntary guarding, since it is impossible for a patient to voluntarily contract a unilateral rectus muscle. It must be emphasized that the only totally reliable finding in acute appendicitis is persistent, localized RLQ pain and tenderness. Even in the absence of a compatible history, anorexia, fever, leukocytosis, or other classic findings, unexplained tenderness in the RLQ is potentially appendicitis until proven otherwise. Failure to adhere to this principle causes an occasional missed diagnosis. Remember, however, that localized abdominal tenderness is frequently absent at the onset and is not specific for acute appendicitis. Classically, the tenderness of appendicitis becomes maximal at McBurney's point, which corresponds to the base of the appendix. This is relatively constant, regardless of where the tip lies. Once the pain is confirmed to be in the RLQ, a few extra minutes are spent examining three or four different areas at random. Each point is palpated, with the inquiry whether it is the site of maximal tenderness. One of the sites is always McBurney's point. In this way the *exact* location of maximal tenderness, if one exists, can be described, rather than using the vague and nondescript term "right lower quadrant tenderness."

Involuntary guarding or rigidity in the RLQ is a sign of peritoneal irritation. Earlier in the course of appendicitis only voluntary guarding may occur. Flexing the patient's knees often allows examination of the abdomen of a patient who is displaying much voluntary guarding (children). Muscular spasm or involuntary guarding is a particularly important local sign, objectively denoting developing peritonitis resulting from progressing parietal peritoneal irritation. An appendix located dorsally or deep in the pelvis may less often induce a local muscular response or tenderness to palpation of the anterior abdominal wall. Failure to realize this fact will lead to delay in operation and a higher perforation rate.

A variety of maneuvers during the physical examination should be performed to elicit the earliest possible manifestation of localized RLQ tenderness because McBurney's point rebound tenderness is the sine qua non of acute appendicitis.

Other Signs

Rovsing's sign is the elicitation of pain in the RLQ during palpation of the left lower quadrant. This is a sign of peritoneal inflammation. As noted previously, Rovsing's sign can be detected by percussion alone on some occasions.

Irritation of the posteriorly located psoas muscle suggests retrocecal inflammation. The *psoas sign* is elicited by having the patient lie on the left side, then slowly extend the right thigh, thereby stretching the iliopsoas muscle and producing pain. Other physicians ask the patient to flex the thigh against the examiner's resistance. If the appendix lies dorsally, near the psoas muscle, the muscle becomes irritated and contracted, causing the patient to flex the hip and knee. Tenderness in the right flank may be noted in patients with retrocecal appendicitis, and therefore a "punch" to this area should be included in the examination in an attempt to define the location of the pain.

A positive obturator sign may occur if the appendix lies near the obturator internus muscle. Pain evoked in the suprapubic area by passive internal and external rotation of the flexed right thigh with the patient supine is a positive test and implies a pelvic location of the appendix.

A vigorous heel slap on the right foot with the leg straight and raised while the patient is supine can transmit vibrations up to the RLQ. If an inflammatory condition like appendicitis exists, the patient may complain of pain. The author has not found this to be a very sensitive test of early localizing acute appendicitis, but others use it reliably. Instead, coughing or the hopping test are more sensitive in the detection of subtle peritonitis.

Cutaneous hyperesthesia of the skin of the abdominal wall in the area supplied by the spinal nerves T-10 to T-12 on the right side has been described in patients with acute appendicitis. Allegedly, the inflammatory condition underlying the area causes increased sensitivity to normal light touch perception, which is interpreted as painful or hypersensitive. This is a curiosity rather than confirmatory in the diagnosis of appendicitis.

Rectal Examination

Rectal examination is necessary in all patients having acute abdominal pain. When the appendix lies deep in the pelvis, anterior abdominal wall findings may be minimal. Loops of small intestine or omentum may limit the spread of inflammation and further minimize the anterior findings. Maximal tenderness may then occur on rectal examination or in the pouch of Douglas. In addition, if perforation and abscess formation has occurred, it may be detected on a rectal examination.

The physical examination should be completed in search of clues that may aid in determining the ultimate cause for the abdominal pain or an extra-abdominal source, since a variety of nonsurgical conditions can mimic appendicitis (see chapter 16).

LABORATORY EVALUATION

Laboratory testing need not be extensive to make the diagnosis of appendicitis. A complete blood count (CBC) usually reveals a modest leukocytosis of 11 000 to 12 000 or up to 16 000 to 17 000. High white blood cell (WBC) counts in excess of 20 000 are usually associated with diffuse peritonitis and perforation or abscess. A high WBC count in the early course of appendicitis is unusual and should lead one to search for an alternative diagnosis. While leukocytosis is common in acute appendicitis, a normal WBC count in no way excludes the diagnosis. In addition, the belief that a normalizing WBC count during active observation indicates that the patient is improving and does not have appendicitis is not valid and results in an occasional missed diagnosis. The CBC should always include a differential. A left shift in the differential, demonstrating more immature forms of leukocytes (bands), is nonspecific but helps confirm that the leukocytosis is the result of an inflammatory condition rather than being an absolute lymphocytosis. This "shift" is probably of more value for diagnostic purposes than the total WBC count.

A urinalysis should be obtained in all patients with abdominal pain, since it is inexpensive and a good screen for other potential disease entities. The absence of blood generally eliminates the possibility of kidney or ureteral stones. Pyuria and bacteriuria have been reported to occur with appendicitis, if the inflamed organ lies on top of the ureter or bladder; however, this is rare, and pyelonephritis or cystitis are the logical diagnoses far more often, given these findings.

Plain radiographs of the abdomen in instances of appendicitis may show a localized ileus, loss of the right psoas border, or an appendicolith. This calcified fecalith, when present and associated with the proper history and physical examination, confirms the diagnosis. However, fecaliths are sufficiently rare on plain radiographs (5%) to make their routine use cost-inefficient. If the history is classic and the physical examination consistent with the diagnosis, do not waste the time or money on a radiograph. On the other hand, if the history is atypical or unavailable or the examination is equivocal, radiographs may be helpful, especially to rule out other diseases. In a female, a pregnancy test should be obtained, not only to exclude pregnancy but for medicolegal precautions before any planned operation.

Beyond these considerations, there is little need for laboratory or radiologic tests in most patients with appendicitis. Barium enema has been used as an aid to the diagnosis. Nonfilling of the appendix on barium enema does not confirm appendicitis but if associated with defacement of the cecum, it is highly suggestive. If the entire length of the appendix fills, the diagnosis is excluded. The overall need for this test is limited, however.

In atypical cases, real-time high-resolution ultrasonography with graded compression may be valuable. The demonstration of a transmural hypoechogenic sausage-shaped structure that is noncompressable and aperistaltic is highly reliable. Additional supportive findings include an appendicolith or a targetlike appearance observed on transverse sections through the appendix. An outer diameter of 7 to 15 mm has been quoted as pathologic. This represents the thick walled organ with its small lumen. Furthermore, ultrasonography may suggest alternative diagnoses in patients with clinically suspected appendicitis. In the presence of pregnancy, ultrasonography is of obvious utility since it obviates radiation exposure. The positive predictive value of ultrasonography in the diagnosis of appendicitis has been 85% to 90%. The use of ultrasonography is not routinely indicated, but in equivocal circumstances, the study may be very helpful.

DIFFERENTIAL DIAGNOSIS

A false-negative appendectomy rate of 15% to 20% has been quoted as still "good surgical practice." In women, even higher false-negative rates are considered acceptable. Removal of a normal appendix on occasion because of unexplained RLQ abdominal pain is more appropriate than a wait-and-see policy, which could result in perforative appendicitis. The usual clinical situation is to make a preoperative diagnosis of acute appendicitis and find a different problem, often also of a surgical nature, or find no explanation for the presentation.

A consideration of other causes of RLQ pain and their subtle differentiation from appendicitis is helpful. Appendicitis can resemble almost any disease that occurs in the abdominal cavity as well as those extraperitoneal problems that produce abdominal symptoms. Familiarity with the following disease entities directs the physician during questioning and examination.

Mesenteric Adenitis
The term mesenteric adenitis implies that inflamed, enlarged mesenteric lymph nodes, especially in the region of the terminal ileum, are the source of the pain and clinical signs and symptoms. Whether this is a distinct clinical

entity or represents the spectrum of another disease process is debatable. Commonly, when the appendix is normal and no other source for RLQ pain can be discovered, mesenteric adenitis is blamed. Clues to the diagnosis include searching for an antecedent upper respiratory infection or otitis media, as these conditions may predate the abdominal pain. Vomiting is not prominent. The fever may be disproportionately high, relative to the findings. Generalized adenopathy may be noted but is uncommon. The pain of mesenteric adenitis starts in the RLQ, rather than midabdominally. The tenderness may not be so well localized as in appendicitis. On occasion, a relative lymphocytosis develops in the differential CBC and probably represents a "viral syndrome"; otherwise, the CBC mimics that of appendicitis. The diagnosis is usually one of exclusion, made at the operating table when the appendix is found to be normal.

Viral or Bacterial Gastroenteritis

Common in childhood, viral or bacterial gastroenteritis is usually associated with profuse diarrhea. Patients with bacterial gastroenteritis tend to be more systemically ill, with fever and chills, but these signs may also occur with the viral form, especially if dehydration has developed. The bowel sounds are hyperactive. Generally, the pain is diffuse but may rarely be localized. Consumption of food tainted with *Staphylococcus* can be associated with explosive diarrhea, abdominal pain, and vomiting, typically occurring 4 to 8 hours after eating. Stool examination for WBCs along with a good history should sort out this diagnosis.

Yersinia Infection

Infection with the organism *Yersinia enterocolitica* or *Y pseudotuberculosis* may occasionally be implicated as the cause of abdominal pain mimicking appendicitis. Pathophysiology relates to the ingestion of the organism from contaminated food. The pathogen is reported to bind preferentially to the mucosa in the region of the terminal ileum. It may in fact be the heretofore unrecognized cause of "mesenteric adenitis." Fever and abdominal pain may be more prominent than diarrhea, although many patients infected with *Yersinia* are asymptomatic. A diversity of other clinical syndromes have been attributed to *Yersinia* such as ileitis, colitis, and acute arthritis. Erythema nodosum, uveitis, or arthritis may be postinfectious complications in a high percentage of patients. In 10% of patients, *Yersinia* may actually be the causative agent of acute appendicitis or it may represent an epiphenomenon. Therefore, the ability to differentiate *Yersinia* infection from acute appendicitis may not be clinically feasible or relevant.

Meckel's Diverticulitis

Meckel's diverticulitis causes clinical signs and symptoms similar to those of appendicitis. The key to being able to make the diagnosis preoperatively is the slightly more medial and cephalad location of the abdominal pain. Most patients with this condition are explored for localizing RLQ pain. When the appendix is found to be normal, routine examination of the distal 2 feet of ileum may reveal the diverticulum.

Intussusception

Intussusception is rare in adults, but it is common in children with abdominal pain. Because an operation is not the first line of therapy, its differentiation has importance. The child is typically less than 2 years old, an age at which appendicitis is uncommon. The child appears well in between attacks of pain, which are manifested as intensive colic, irritability, vomiting, and drawing the legs up to the abdomen. A radiograph of the abdomen is sometimes helpful in the evaluation of abdominal pain in the very young and in this setting may reveal an obstructive pattern.

Regional Enteritis (Crohn's Disease)

Often a patient has a history of regional enteritis, or someone in the patient's family has had it. The pain and clinical symptoms may mimic appendicitis exactly, except diarrhea may be a prominent part of the history. Often, without this information, operation is unavoidable. Remove the appendix only if the cecum and appendix are free of the underlying inflammatory bowel disease.

Perforated Ulcer

A perforated ulcer can mimic appendicitis if the spilled gastric or duodenal contents run exclusively down to the RLQ. This is a rare and uncommon presentation of perforated ulcer. The history should aid in the diagnosis, and a known past ulcer diathesis should be sought. In most patients with perforated ulcer, the occurrence of the pain tends to be very acute, with severe onset noted immediately, in contradistinction to the pain of acute appendicitis. Abdominal tenderness and peritonitis with a rigid or "boardlike" abdomen occur early in the presentation. This atypical history for appendicitis should prompt abdominal radiography, which usually reveals free air.

Diverticular Disease of the Colon

A redundant left colon with diverticulitis lying in the RLQ may be challenging to distinguish from appendicitis. Sigmoid diverticulitis has been called "left-sided appendicitis," since the symptoms can mimic appendicitis so closely. A perforated cecal diverticulum is difficult, if not impossible, to differentiate. The peak incidence of the disease is in an older age group, but many younger people are discovered to have perforated diverticulitis, thus leading to confusion. Change in bowel habits, occult blood in the stool, or a palpable mass may be detected. Diarrhea may accompany diverticulitis more often than it does appendicitis. The leukocytosis tends to be higher than in appendicitis.

Carcinoma of the Ascending or Sigmoid Colon

A perforative or obstructive carcinoma located in the ascending colon or the redundant sigmoid may mimic the pain of appendicitis. The patient population tends to be older and, as with diverticulitis, there may be a change of bowel habits. Weight loss may have occurred. Occult blood in the stool or a hypochromic anemia may be detected and should heighten the suspicion. A physical examination may disclose a mass. In the elderly population, a low-pressure barium enema may be needed prior to laparotomy to exclude these possibilities.

Torsion of an Epiploic Appendage

Torsion with subsequent infarction of these fatty appendages to the colon can mimic appendicitis. The history tends to be atypical, with the patient appearing less sick and only complaining of localized abdominal pain. Shift in the pain pattern is unusual and should be an important clue, at least differentiating it from appendicitis. The CBC tends to be normal. Operation may be unavoidable if the symptoms do not resolve.

Urinary Tract Infection

Pyelonephritis on the right side may mimic retrocecal appendicitis, since the physical findings predominate in the flank. The patient has high fever, chills, and rigor, and an abnormal urinalysis with bacteriuria. Although microscopic hematuria and pyuria are reported to occur if the inflamed appendix overlies the ureter or bladder, this is rare. Cystitis is usually evidenced by intense dysuria and urinary frequency without associated chills and rigors. The history, physical findings, and skillful interpretation of a urine sediment should lead to the correct diagnosis.

Perinephric Abscess

Patients usually have a more insidious course, with high fevers and rigors, which is uncommon in acute appendicitis. Because marked costovertebral angle pain and tenderness predominate, the confusion with retrocecal appendicitis is understandable. A perinephric abscess will often produce a reflex ileus with vomiting and the associated findings of plain radiography. Overall, these patients appear much more systemically ill. The prodrome associated with appendicitis is absent.

Ureteral Stone

A migrating calculus in the right ureter can mimic appendicitis. A history of previous stones may be obtainable. Most patients have hematuria, and this should be ascertained in any patient prior to planned appendectomy. The pain may radiate to the ipsilateral testis or vulva and is a diagnostic clue. Urinary frequency may be one of the symptoms. The pain is often extremely severe and associated with profuse vomiting, both of which are atypical for appendicitis.

Rectus Sheath Hematoma or Rupture

A hematoma or rupture of the rectus sheath may be confused with appendicitis, but the history should serve to differentiate this. Rupture of the rectus usually follows exertion, such as straining or lifting weights, severe coughing, trauma, or pregnancy. Hematomas usually occur in patients on anticoagulants. Carnett's test may be helpful in differentiating abdominal wall tenderness from intra-abdominal tenderness. This test is performed with the patient supine. The abdomen is palpated to elicit tenderness or a mass. If such an area is found, the patient is then asked to elevate his or her head, thus contracting the recti. A persistent mass or tenderness implies an abdominal wall location, since tense recti will protect intra-abdominal pathologic lesions from being detected. Ultrasound or computed tomography (CT) can be diagnostic.

Neutropenic Colitis

Neutropenic colitis is a fulminant, necrotizing process of the terminal ileum, cecum, or ascending colon occurring in immunocompromised patients, especially those rendered neutropenic from chemotherapy. Abdominal pain with localization near McBurney's point, abdominal distention, diarrhea, and fever are prominent features. The illness progresses to full-blown sepsis dramatically and quickly if untreated. Surgical mortality is approximately 50%. Abdominal plain radiographs occasionally reveal pneumatosis of the right colon, but diagnosis is based on clinical findings in the neutropenic patient.

Acute Cholecystitis

Acute cholecystitis can mimic appendicitis, since both are accompanied by pain on the right side, fever, and vomiting. Antecedent anorexia is usually not present because the attack of cholecystitis is usually precipitated by a meal. An inflamed gallbladder will frequently descend to the right mid or lower abdomen and then become palpable, unless the patient is obese.

Respiratory Diseases

Pneumonia, pleurisy, and influenza can present with clinical signs and symptoms resembling acute appendicitis: pain, tenderness, and guarding in the right side of the abdomen. Lobar pneumonia in children will commonly present with fever and abdominal pain. Therefore, a chest radiograph is essential before operative intervention in any patient in whom appendicitis is suspected. A cough, shortness of breath, or productive sputum may be noted. Auscultory findings may or may not be present over the lung fields. Leukocyte counts tend to be higher than in appendicitis.

Viral Hepatitis

Viral hepatitis can be associated with abdominal pain, nausea, and anorexia. As a rule, however, the pain does not localize in the RLQ. Once jaundice is manifested, the confusion clears.

Gastritis

Gastritis produces epigastric pain, which can also be the initial symptom of acute appendicitis. However, serial examination shows lack of migration to the RLQ. Drugs implicated in gastritis should be sought in the history.

Psoas Abscess

A psoas abscess may cause irritation of the iliopsoas muscle and produce findings identical to a retrocecal perforative appendix. A psoas abscess is usually secondary to some other process, one of which can be appendicitis.

Ruptured Aortic Aneurysm

A rupturing aortic abdominal aneurysm can produce pain in the lower mid-abdomen, back, and hips. The pain is usually severe, sudden in onset, and there may be associated shock. A pulsatile mass should be palpable near the umbilicus if the patient is not obese. Otherwise the abdomen may reveal mild diffuse tenderness or peritonitis from the irritating blood. Femoral pulses may be diminished. If the rupture is contained and the patient is obese, the diagnosis can prove difficult. Often there is a history of vascular disease and a male predominance. Cross-table abdominal plain radiographs may reveal an expanded, calcified aortic wall displaced toward the left side, with loss of the psoas shadow.

Foreign-Body Perforation

Although most ingested foreign bodies pass spontaneously, perforation of the gastrointestinal tract may occur. Sharp objects such as fish or chicken bones or toothpicks may be ingested by young children, alcoholic, or psychiatric patients or, more commonly, edentulous individuals with diminished oral sensitivity. The history of ingesting a sharp object is usually absent, however, making the diagnosis difficult. The ileocecal region is the most common site of perforation. Acute peritonitis may develop, requiring operation, or vague chronic obstructive symptoms may occur over the course of several days or weeks. Typically the small hole seals and a phlegmon or abscess forms near the perforation. The patient may feel reasonably well except for a fever, localized abdominal pain, and a mass. Laparotomy will reveal the resulting inflammatory problem, but often the exact cause of the perforation remains enigmatic.

Disorders of the Female Reproductive Tract

Pelvic Inflammatory Disease. Pelvic inflammatory disease (PID) can be acute salpingitis, a tubo-ovarian abscess, or a hydrosalpinx. These conditions are probably responsible for the most confusion with acute appendicitis. All produce pain below the umbilicus migrating to the pelvis and are commonly accompanied by nausea and vomiting. Anorexia may or may not be present.

PID is often associated with a high fever (101° to 102° F) and tachycardia. The salpingitis associated with PID is usually bilateral, but unilateral involvement, especially with associated pyosalpinx, does occur. A pelvic examination usually reveals bilateral tenderness, especially with cervical motion and vaginal discharge, which should always be Gram's stained in search of *Gonococcus* and cultured for *Chlamydia*. The infection typically is recurrent and tends to occur within 7 days of the most recent menstrual period. Sexual promiscuity should also be ascertained in the history.

Ruptured Follicular or Corpus Luteum Cyst. It may be difficult to distinguish a ruptured follicular from a ruptured corpus luteum cyst. The pain of ovulation caused by a follicular cyst can be quite similar to that of acute appendicitis. There may be associated bleeding with ovulation and, if severe enough, it will irritate the diaphragm and refer pain to a shoulder (Kehr's sign). Occurrence of the pain at about midpoint of the menstrual cycle should help with the diagnosis, and during 12 to 16 hours of observation, most patients improve. The pain usually starts acutely in the RLQ rather than exhibiting the slow prodrome associated with appendicitis. This is an important differentiating point. The patients are typically younger than 25 years and may have a history of painful ovulation. The pain of a ruptured corpus luteum cyst occurs near the onset of menses. The WBC count typically is normal or is minimally elevated and there is usually no shift in the differential.

Ectopic Pregnancy. Establishing the diagnosis of ectopic pregnancy remains challenging. More than 80% of these pregnancies occur in the fallopian tube. A history of previous ectopic pregnancy is an important risk factor, as is pelvic infection, previous induced abortion, use of an intrauterine device, endometriosis, and previous tubal sterilization. Pelvic or abdominal pain is the chief complaint in more than 90% of patients. Abnormal uterine bleeding occurs 50% to 80% of the time, but clinical shock is rare. Amenorrhea may or may not be present but is important to note. A physical examination may be most remarkable for adnexal tenderness and a mass. Transvaginal high-resolution ultrasonography may demonstrate an extrauterine gestational sac; however, findings tend to be nonspecific. Radioimmunoassay of the beta subunit of HCG is positive in more than 95% of patients. This sensitive test becomes positive 9 to 10 days after ovulation if pregnancy occurs. Diagnostic laparoscopy may be required to make the diagnosis of ectopic pregnancy.

Adnexal Torsion. Adnexal torsion most commonly involves the ovary and distal half of the fallopian tube. It is a diseased or cystic ovary that usually results in torsion. The pain and vomiting come on simultaneously and tend to be worse than with appendicitis. The pain is usually severe, acute, and localized at the onset. A bimanual pelvic examination reveals tenderness in excess of that anticipated with appendicitis. The abdominal examination is notable for rebound tenderness. Torsion may result in a compromised blood supply to the affected side, with resultant infarction and gangrene.

Pedunculated Myomas. Pedunculated myomas have the propensity to rotate on their pedicle and cause pain. This is difficult to distinguish from appendicitis, if it occurs on the right side. The severity of the pain is similar to tubo-ovarian torsion. The patients appear more uncomfortable earlier in the course of their illness, and the prodrome of appendicitis is absent.

Endometriosis. Dysmenorrhea caused by endometriosis can induce localized pain and tenderness. This may present with physical findings identical to appendicitis and, in fact, endometriosis has been reported to involve the appendix; however, this is rare and usually asymptomatic. Unless the patient gives the history of known endometriosis or cyclical pain, the diagnosis will be difficult without operative intervention.

Disorders of the Male Reproductive Tract
The physician must remember to perform a thorough genital examination and search for hernias on the disrobed patient.

Seminal Vesiculitis. Seminal vesiculitis may produce diffuse lower abdominal pain but, typically, without localization. Nausea, vomiting, and a high fever and chills may be noted. Rectal examination reveals marked tenderness in the area of the prostate.

Torsion of the Testes. Testicular torsion leads to severe pain, similar to renal colic. Vomiting often occurs. When this diagnosis is missed, it is generally because of omission of the testicular examination. Contusion or tumor of the testicle can present with apparent RLQ pain, but the physical examination should quickly sort out the real cause.

Epididymitis. The hemiscrotum is usually very tender and the inflamed epididymis can readily be palpated.

Malingering
A malingering patient often presents describing recurrent vague or even localized abdominal pain. The symptoms tend to be chronic and recurrent. Often these patients are quite knowledgeable about medical and surgical illnesses and use appropriate jargon from having read about their "disease." If the history and findings are atypical, further evaluation is indicated. Subtle maneuvers to elicit true RLQ tenderness (like the use of the palpatory stethoscope, mentioned above) may uncover the malingerer. Alternatively, the patient must be given the benefit of the doubt, and unexplained RLQ tenderness will likely lead to intervention. Recurrent abdominal pain in the child can be

a vexing problem and in the absence of objective findings or laboratory analysis, a search for a social problem is appropriate.

SPECIAL SITUATIONS

Appendicitis in the Very Young

Fewer than 2% of all children treated for appendicitis are younger than 3 years old. In this age group, appendicitis is a more serious disease than in adolescents because the perforation rate is high and in some series approaches 90%. Furthermore, it is estimated that up to one third of patients will have sought medical attention prior to perforation. Diagnostic accuracy is diminished because of atypical features and lack of effective communication skills. The parents are often the only source of the history. In children, anorexia may be absent and vomiting and diarrhea more common. Since gastroenteritis is also common, loose stools add confusion to the picture. Frequently, it helps to ask if other siblings also have a diarrhealike illness. A history of midabdominal pain migrating to the RLQ is uncommon.

An accurate physical examination is difficult in the irritable infant. Many children are apprehensive of physicians, since they feel threatened or fear a painful examination. Allowing the parent to hold the child may facilitate the examination. A hurried examination causing pain provides unreliable findings; therefore developing rapport is worth the time spent. The best assessment of tenderness is revealed in the child's face rather than through palpation and repetitively asking where it hurts most. The classic test to elicit rebound tenderness, performed by suddenly releasing a deeply palpating hand, will overestimate the incidence of peritonitis in a child and is not recommended. Better methods are the subtle maneuvers described previously, such as percussion tenderness. Localized RLQ tenderness is often not ascertainable. Children commonly have diffuse abdominal pain and without the appendix being perforated. Rectal examination in children tends to be traumatic and usually does not offer much in diagnostic yield. Ultimately, dehydration, lethargy, high fever or hypothermia, and abdominal distention ensue, and the diagnosis of appendicitis is entertained.

Abdominal plain radiographs may be helpful in the young child and infant. If a fecalith is identified in the proper clinical setting, it is generally pathognomonic. Free air associated with perforative appendicitis is a rarity (reported 0% to 7%) and should not be sought.

Appendicitis in the Elderly

Appendicitis in the elderly is a more serious disorder when compared to other age groups. Fortunately, the prevalence of the disease among the aged is low. This rapidly growing segment of the population constitutes the majority of the deaths from appendicitis, usually as a result of concomitant health problems and delay in diagnosis. Recollection for the details in the history may be impaired because of failing memory. Often the patients ascribe their symptoms to chronic disease. The physical findings may be vague or masked as patients present late in the course of their illness. Abdominal distention may be the only sign in some patients.

The elderly, for a variety of reasons, may have a blunted response to infection, resulting in lack of fever or leukocytosis. Radiographs often disclose an ileus or obstructive pattern. The surgeon faced with indolent, atypical symptoms in patients with other medical problems is hesitant to intervene. The barium enema and ultrasonography may have their greatest use in these perplexing patients.

Appendicitis in Pregnant Women

Acute appendicitis is the most common extrauterine surgical emergency with a reported incidence of 0.38 and 1.41 per 1000 pregnancies; however, the actual incidence of appendicitis is not increased. Diagnosis is more difficult, especially after the first trimester. This is because anorexia, nausea, vomiting, and vague abdominal pain are frequent with pregnancy. Palpation of the abdomen is considerably more difficult with an enlarging uterus. Guarding and rebound are less constant because of the laxity of the abdominal wall musculature. The diagnosis of acute appendicitis in pregnancy is further complicated by the alteration in location of the cecum and appendix. In 1932, Baer studied 78 pregnant women with barium enemas and noted the degree of appendiceal displacement. After the third month of gestation the appendix began to be displaced above McBurney's point. By the eighth month, 93% of the women were found to have their appendices above the iliac crest and 80% displayed an upward rotation of the base from the horizontal plane. In general, there is a counterclockwise rotation, with the tip of the appendix being displaced cephalad. Therefore the location of maximal tenderness can change, depending on the stage of the pregnancy. In addition, the ability of the omentum to migrate to the RLQ is impaired in pregnancy, and this results in a higher incidence of diffuse peritonitis. A useful sign may be to roll the patient on her left side. If the pain shifts, it is likely in the uterus. If the pain remains in the RLQ, it is more likely appendicitis. Laboratory data may be less helpful because a mild leukocytosis, often seen with appendicitis, is normal during pregnancy. However, a left shift in the differential is not expected in uncomplicated pregnancy.

Often the physician is reluctant to operate because of the patient's pregnancy and the fear of inducing labor and of fetal loss. This is a grave error and has led to a reported perforation rate of 25%. The best rule is to treat the patient as if she were not pregnant. Once perforation occurs, labor may ensue, resulting in prematurity or fetal demise. Peritonitis leads to increased fetal loss, which has been quoted to be 35% to 70%. Women between the 24th to 36th week of gestation who undergo appendectomy have a clear excess of premature deliveries within the week after the operation (almost 25%). There may also be a higher incidence of lower-birth-weight infants in those patients who have undergone appendectomy during pregnancy.

Babler's statement from the early 1900s is apt today: "The mortality of appendicitis complicating pregnancy is the mortality of delay."

Postoperative Appendicitis

Acute appendicitis, which occurs within a short period of time after another abdominal operation, is rare and difficult to diagnose. Retrospectively, most patients follow a typical pattern. Confusion predominates, however, since prospectively the symptoms are consistent with the postoperative findings of many patients after abdominal operations. Normally administered narcotics may alter pain recognition. Antibiotics may inhibit the inflammatory response. Therefore, delay predominates in the clinical pattern. RLQ pain, tenderness, and guarding is a consistent finding and should not be ignored, especially when the site of surgery was distant from that region. Because of these difficulties in diagnosis, some surgeons advocate routine incidental appendectomy. However, because postoperative appendicitis occurs in only 0.1% of all instances of acute appendicitis, this does not seem justified.

Chronic Appendicitis

Appendiceal luminal obstruction resulting from a soft fecalith or lymphoid hypertrophy may resolve spontaneously. Whether this occurs and leads to chronic or recurrent appendicitis is controversial. In these situations the history may be atypical, the physical findings mild and improving, and laboratory data normal. These patients are often discharged with a diagnosis of mesenteric adenitis or a viral syndrome. Weeks, months, or years later the symptoms may recur. The temptation to remove the appendix for the reason of chronic appendicitis should be resisted. Often the source of the pain requires further delineation, and appendectomy does not lead to a satisfactory resolution of pain in most patients. Some patients' conditions are improved by appendectomy, and pathologic examination of the organ reveals fibrosis and chronic inflammation. No clear guidelines are available for the management of patients who fall into this category. The increased use of laparoscopy may be diagnostically helpful in this situation. Mucoceles of the appendix, on the other hand, will often present with a vague history of chronic lower abdominal pain. This process is characterized by accumulated mucus in a distended appendix. Mucosal hyperplasia can lead to mucocele formation, with obstruction of the lumen and distention of the appendix and resultant pain. Pressure within the lumen then may overcome the obstruction leading to discharge of the mucus into the colonic lumen with relief of pain. Mucoceles are often palpable or easily demonstrated with ultrasonography.

Missed Appendicitis

Perforation may occur as soon as 6 hours after the onset of the symptoms of appendicitis, but it usually occurs 24 to 48 hours after symptoms begin. If peritonitis occurs, the patient presents with an acute abdomen. However, the appendix can perforate and be contained by omentum, loops of small intestine, or the retroperitoneum. Typically these patients will present with an obscure history, often having been evaluated in an emergency department and sent home with a diagnosis of gastroenteritis or urinary tract infection. Instead they now may or may not be febrile and have RLQ fullness or a mass with tenderness, guarding, and pain. The mass in the RLQ may represent an abscess cavity or the omentum wrapped around an inflamed, perforated appendix. Frequently they have been eating and conducting normal daily activities without knowledge of the underlying pathologic conditions. Confirming the diagnosis is the first task. In these confusing situations, ultrasonography, barium enema, and CT may be helpful. If an abscess is identified, management is controversial, and the trend is toward percutaneous drainage and interval appendectomy. This decision is obviously based upon the patient's clinical condition.

SUGGESTED READING

Barr D, van Heerden JA, Mucha P. The diagnostic challenge of postoperative acute appendicitis. *World J Surg.* 1991; 15:526.

Bennion RS, Thompson JE, Gil J, et al. The role of *Yersinia enterocolitica* in appendicitis in the southwestern United States. *Am Surg.* 1991; 57:766.

Mahoodian S. Appendicitis complicating pregnancy. *South Med J.* 1992; 85:19.

Mazze RI, Kallen B. Appendectomy during pregnancy: a Swedish Registry study of 778 cases. *Obstet Gynecol.* 1991; 77:835.

Neblett WW, Pietsch JB, Holcomb GW. Acute abdominal conditions in children and adolescents. *Surg Clin North Am.* 1988; 68:415.

Rajagopalan AE, Mason JH, Kennedy M, et al. The value of the barium enema in the diagnosis of acute appendicitis. *Arch Surg.* 1977; 112:531.

Savrin RA, Clausen K, Martin EW, et al. Chronic and recurrent appendicitis. *Am J Surg.* 1979; 137:355.

Shen GH, Wong R, Daller J, et al. Does the retrocecal position of the vermiform appendix alter the clinical course of acute appendicitis? *Arch Surg.* 1991; 126:569.

Skaane P, Amland PF, Nordshus T, et al. Ultrasonography in patients with suspected acute appendicitis: a prospective study. *Br J Radiol.* 1990; 63:787.

Storer EH. Appendix. In: Schwartz SI, ed. *Principles of Surgery.* 5th ed. New York, NY: McGraw-Hill Book Co Inc; 1989.

Waxman K, Mason GR. Appendicitis and Appendiceal Abscess. In: Nyhus LM, Baker RJ, eds. *Mastery of Surgery.* 2nd ed. Boston, Mass: Little, Brown & Co, 1992.

CHAPTER 6

■

Biliary Tract Disease

Joseph Kokoszka, MD
Joseph M. Vitello, MD

In the evaluation of upper abdominal pain, biliary tract disease in one form or another must be considered in the differential diagnosis. It is the purpose of this chapter to review the pertinent anatomy and physiology and describe how this knowledge, along with a history and physical examination, can assist the clinician in making the correct diagnosis.

ANATOMY AND PHYSIOLOGY

The gallbladder is a pear-shaped organ attached to the inferior surface of the liver. Normally it is capable of storing 50 mL of bile and up to 300 mL if obstructed. The relationship of the gallbladder to adjacent organs may help explain the varied presentations of acute cholecystitis. The most distal aspect of the gallbladder is in contact with the anterior abdominal wall just inferior to the costal margin. The anterior surface of the body of the gallbladder adheres to the liver by connective tissue, and the posterior surface is in direct contact with the transverse colon and duodenum. The gallbladder empties via the cystic duct into the common hepatic duct, at which point it becomes the common bile duct (CBD). The CBD continues posterior to the duodenum and head of the pancreas to enter the duodenum via the ampulla of Vater. The critical anatomy of the biliary tree occurs within Calot's triangle, that area bordered by the cystic duct, the common hepatic duct, and the cystic artery. (Many authors have expanded this triangle to include the inferior edge of the liver rather than the cystic artery, as originally described by Calot).

Active secretion of bile by both hepatocytes and cells lining the biliary tree are responsible for the production of 500 to 1500 mL of bile each day. The bile flows from both the left and right hepatic ducts into the confluence, the common hepatic duct. From here it flows unimpeded into the duodenum. Between meals the sphincter of Oddi is closed and bile flows into the gallbladder, where it is stored and concentrated. In response to a fatty meal, cholecystokinin (CCK) is released from the small intestine and serves as the stimulus for gallbladder contraction and for relaxation of the sphincter of Oddi.

DIAGNOSIS

History

Acute cholecystitis is defined as acute inflammation of the gallbladder, usually as a result of obstruction of the cystic duct by a stone, with signs ranging from mild edema and congestion to severe infection with gangrene and perforation.

Acute cholecystitis begins with abdominal pain of acute onset that gradually increases in severity over time. The pain typically occurs after a meal, in contradistinction to the pain of peptic ulcer disease, which tends to occur and is worsened by the fasting state. In the classic situation, the meal is high in fat content, deep-fried, or spicy. This is by no means consistently true, however, and in fact, the pain may occur in the fasting state or after ingestion of a bland meal. A number of patients will be awakened from sleep with the pain. Initially, most victims of acute cholecystitis blame "heartburn" or "indigestion" for their symptoms. The progressive, constant pain, which may last 6 to 12 hours before relenting, is often a diagnostic clue to differentiate acute from chronic cholecystitis. The pain is located in the right subcostal region but may originate in the epigastric area and subsequently localize to the right upper quadrant (RUQ). At times the pain may be referred or radiate around to the back and right scapula. As many as 60% to 75% of patients will admit to having previous similar episodes of pain that subsided spontaneously. Distention of the gallbladder may include nausea and vomiting during an attack of cholecystitis. The vomiting is rarely as severe as with intestinal obstruction, and metabolic derangements seldom occur.

Certain populations are known to be at increased risk of gallstone development and subsequently cholecystitis. This includes cirrhotics and those with hemolytic diseases, where the increased bilirubin load predisposes the individual to the formation of pigment (bilirubinate) calculi. Cholesterol stones are more common in Native Americans, as well, and in those people who fit into the classic four Fs of cholelithiasis (fat, female, fertile, forty). Although gallstone disease is not exclusively limited to these groups, this stratification may help in the initial evaluation.

Physical Examination

A patient with acute cholecystitis can present in moderate distress secondary to the abdominal pain. A low-grade temperature (99° to 100°F) is the norm, and higher temperatures or a more toxic appearance of the patient should suggest a more complicated disease process. Mild tachycardia induced by the ongoing inflammatory process may also be detected. Scleral icterus may be noted, but in the majority of instances of acute cholecystitis, the serum bilirubin is not elevated.

Abdominal examination may reveal mild distention caused by a reactive ileus secondary to the inflammation. Bowel sounds tend to be normal without high pitches, rushes, or tinkling. Tenderness in the RUQ remains one of the most common and reliable signs in the diagnosis of acute cholecystitis. At times the tenderness may even be present in the epigastrium. In one third of the patients a palpable gallbladder is present. Obesity and voluntary guarding of the abdominal wall musculature may prevent detection of the distended gallbladder in the remainder. With the induction of general anesthesia and abdominal wall relaxation, the opportunity presents itself to reexamine the patient in search of a palpable gallbladder. When the gallbladder is markedly distended it may become inferiorly displaced into the right midabdomen. This is occasionally a source of diagnostic confusion, as the patient appears to have right lower quadrant pain. By starting the abdominal palpation in the right lower quadrant and slowly advancing to the RUQ, this confusion is usually eliminated. Inspiratory arrest during deep palpation of the RUQ (Murphy's sign) may be elicited in acute cholecystitis but is not specific for the disease. Inflammatory conditions of the liver (hepatitis, abscess) or space-occupying lesions (adenomas, metastatic carcinoma) will also produce this finding. Acute cholecystitis may be associated with cutaneous hyperesthesias in the right subscapular area (Boas' sign), although this finding is inconsistent.

Laboratory Evaluation

Since acute cholecystitis is an inflammatory process, a mild leukocytosis with a left shift is often observed. The usual range is 12 000 to 15 000; elevations greater than this should raise suspicion that a complication of acute cholecystitis has occurred (gangrene, perforation).

Irritation of the cystic duct either from the impacted gallstone or associated inflammation in and around Calot's triangle may cause an elevation of the alkaline phosphatase. Because of the anatomic proximity, stasis or even obstruction of the CBD can occur in acute cholecystitis, resulting in mild elevation of the serum bilirubin to 2 to 3mg/dL. The bilirubin rises relatively late when compared to the alkaline phosphatase. Levels of bilirubin greater than 3mg/dL should raise suspicion of choledocholithiais.

Diagnostic Imaging

Plain Radiography. The use of standard plain radiographs (ie, kidney, ureter, and bladder [KUB], flat plate of the abdomen, and obstructive series) may be useful for the overall evaluation of the acute abdomen but is of limited value in the diagnosis of acute cholecystitis or cholelithiasis. Only 15% of gallstones contain enough calcium to make them radiopaque and visible on these studies. Other findings related to biliary diseases that may be seen on conventional roentgenograms include calcification of the gallbladder wall (porcelain gallbladder) or calcium-saturated bile (milk of calcium). Occasionally, cholesterol gallstones may contain air trapped within their centers, producing a characteristic appearance of the so-called "Mercedes-Benz sign."

Air outlining the gallbladder, so called emphysematous cholecystitis, suggests there is a serious bacterial infection producing the gas that defines the gallbladder wall. This finding should prompt urgent surgical intervention and microbiologic evaluation in search of gram-positive rods, which may suggest a clostridial infection. Air within the biliary tree produces a change in relative densities and may be visualized on conventional radiographs. This finding may indicate a previous enterobiliary anastomosis or a serious complication of cholelithiasis or cholecystitis, including cholecystoenteric fistula and resultant gallstone ileus or a gas-forming bacterial infection within the gallbladder.

Oral Cholecystography. The oral cholecystogram (OCG), introduced in 1924 by Cole and Graham, was the first diagnostic procedure able to document the presence of cholelithiasis. The patient is required to take a number (4 to 12) of contrast-containing tablets (tryoppanoate or iopanoic acid) in the evening, 14 to 17 hours prior to the test. The fasting patient then receives abdominal radiography the following morning. The tablets must be absorbed by the small intestine and the contrast enter the hepatic circulation for the test to work properly. Provided the gastrointestinal, enterohepatic, and biliary systems are functional, any gallstones present can be seen on subsequent conventional abdominal radiographs. The gallstones appear as filling defects that move in response to positional changes of the patient. A double dose, nonvisualized gallbladder is a good functional test, implies cystic duct obstruction, and is an indication for cholecystectomy. Because of the complex interplay of systems, a significant number of false-negative examinations occur with the OCG. Reasons for this include patient noncompliance in taking the pills, emesis, malabsorption, hepatic dysfunction, hyperbilirubinemia (>3mg/dL), and pancreatitis. The utility of the OCG is further limited by the time interval required for the test to be performed.

Ultrasonography. Real-time ultrasonography has evolved to become the test of choice in the diagnosis of acute cholecystitis. Ultrasonography is able to provide a safe, rapid, noninvasive, and inexpensive method to evaluate the biliary system. Although the test is most commonly performed in the radiology department, portable ultrasonographic units allow the examination to be performed at the bedside for patients too ill to be transported. An anatomic image of the gallbladder and biliary tree can be seen with ultrasonography as well as adjacent structures (pancreas, liver, kidney). This offers an advantage over other biliary imaging techniques, especially if the patient proves not to have gallstones, since the ultrasonogram may uncover another source of the symptoms. Gallstones appear as hypoechoic shadows on the ultrasonogram. The presence of a gallstone lodged in the cystic duct is diagnostic for acute calculous cholecystitis. Associated findings that may suggest acute cholecystitis include thickening of the gallbladder wall, dilatation of the biliary radicles, and the presence of pericholecystic fluid. Tenderness over the gallbladder during the ultrasonographic examination is called the ultrasonic Murphy's sign and is present in 85% of patients with acute cholecystitis.

The test can be limited if the acoustic window needed to perform this examination is obscured by overlying bowel gas or fat in the excessively obese patient. In experienced hands, an accuracy rate of 98% is possible in diagnosing acute cholecystitis.

Gallbladder Scintigraphy. A relatively rapid and safe test for the diagnosis of acute cholecystitis is the HIDA scan. Unlike ultrasonography, the HIDA is able to provide information about both the anatomy and physiology of the biliary system.

A technetium-labeled derivative of iminodiacetic acid is injected intravenously and is metabolized by the hepatocyte. The radionuclide is then excreted into the biliary system. Images are obtained at 10- to 15-minute intervals for 1 to 2 hours. A normal study will show uptake of the radionuclide within 5 minutes. Unobstructed flow of bile will allow the bile ducts to be visualized at 45 minutes, with subsequent duodenal filling at 60 minutes. Failure of the gallbladder to fill with radionuclide after duodenal visualization is evidence of cystic duct obstruction (ie, most commonly, acute cholecystitis). However, most literature suggests waiting up to 4 hours, since filling of the gallbladder may be delayed.

The HIDA has an accuracy of 94% in diagnosing acute cholecystitis. This test cannot detect the presence or absence of gallstones as the ultrasonogram can. However, patients who cannot be adequately evaluated with ultrasonography (lack of acoustic window because of obesity or overlying bowel gas) can be examined with HIDA. False-positive examinations may occur in patients who have been on restricted oral intake for prolonged periods or in alcoholics. Since the iminodiacetic acid has a stronger affinity for the bile than the oral agents used in the OCG, it can be used with reliability in patients with bilirubin levels greater than 10mg/dL.

Endoscopic Retrograde Cholangiopancreatography. Endoscopic retrograde cholangiopancreatography (ERCP) is a minimally invasive test that is able to delineate the biliary tree and at times serve as a therapeutic maneuver. It is a technically demanding test that requires an endoscopist skilled in this technique. A side-viewing endoscope is passed orally to the ampulla of Vater; the ampulla is cannulated, and contrast is injected under fluoroscopic guidance. Visualization of the papilla is successful in 80% to 90% of patients. The biliary tree, as well as any filling defects, can be identified in this manner.

In addition to its being diagnostic, the endoscope permits therapeutic procedures such as removal of distal ductal stones or sphincterotomy to be performed through it.

ERCP is associated with a 5% complication rate, which is much higher than other diagnostic maneuvers. Possible complications include bleeding, pancreatitis, sepsis, and cholangitis. The cost to perform this examination is markedly higher than that of other tests.

Percutaneous Transhepatic Cholangiography. In percutaneous transhepatic cholangiography (PTC) a needle placed percutaneously is inserted into an intrahepatic bile duct under ultrasonic guidance. The needle placement is confirmed by the ability to aspirate bile through the needle, at which point radiopaque contrast is injected under fluoroscopic guidance. The proximal biliary tree is opacified, and any filling defects are identified. The PTC does not require as much skill to perform as does ERCP, but the risks of bleeding, cholangitis, and pancreatitis also exist.

DISORDERS OF THE BILIARY TRACT

Chronic Cholecystitis

The pathogenesis of the symptoms in this clinical entity is due to transient obstruction of the cystic duct by a calculus but without the associated inflammation found in acute cholecystitis. These patients tend to have recurrent attacks resulting from the presence of numerous gallstones. Typically, two symptoms predominate in chronic cholecystitis, biliary colic and dyspepsia.

The definition of colic is a pain with a spasmodic and episodic nature lasting for a brief period, the classic example of which is renal colic. Biliary colic differs because the pain is steady and gradually increases over time (about 1 hour to plateau). Once the pain reaches the plateau it may remain at that intensity for several hours and slowly relent. Thus the term *biliary colic* is really a misnomer. The pain is located in the RUQ and may radiate to either the back or subscapular region. Biliary colic is the presenting symptom in 75% of patients with chronic calculous cholecystitis. The second described symptom, dyspepsia, encompasses a number of rather vague, nonspecific complaints. This may include fatty-food intolerance, flatulence, eructation, and postprandial bloating. One or more of these symptoms is present in 80% of the affected population.

Physical examination of these patients tends to be unremarkable. Fever is notably absent when compared to acute cholecystitis. Some patients may have RUQ tenderness on deep palpation, but Murphy's sign is not elicited. Similarly, laboratory tests tend to be normal, most notably the white blood count (WBC). The diagnosis of cholelithiasis is confirmed with either ultrasonography or OCG.

The differentiation of acute cholecystitis from chronic, symptomatic cholelithiasis has much clinical importance (Table 8). Patients will commonly present to the emergency department with abdominal pain and a known history of gallstones or have calculi identified during evaluation of their pain. The acutely ill patient warrants admission to the hospital and probably cholecystectomy during this setting. The chronic cholecystitis patient may be given a follow-up appointment in the clinic or office to discuss elective cholecystectomy, which often involves only a 23-hour hospital stay.

Acute Acalculous Cholecystitis

Whereas in acute cholecystitis the implied initiating agents are gallstones, no specific agents have been identified in acute acalculous cholecystitis. The common factor in this disease is the absence of stones upon ultrasound examination. Multifactorial events are most likely responsible for acute acalculous cholecystitis. These include: biliary stasis secondary to ampullary spasm, decreased emptying of the gallbladder as a result of fasting, edema of the cystic duct, and dehydration, which increases the viscosity of bile.

This clinical entity is characteristically seen in patients with multiple medical problems, namely sepsis, severe burns, trauma, and those patients on parenteral alimentation without enteral stimulation. This group of patients already has an inherently high mortality rate; thus it becomes imperative to make the diagnosis of acalculous cholecystitis quickly, since it is associated with a mortality of greater than 50%.

The presenting signs and symptoms of acute acalculous cholecystitis can be the same as those of calculous cholecystitis, but at times the only presentation may be sepsis of unknown origin. However, the patients in whom this condition most commonly occurs are often unable to provide a history. In addition if the patient is sedated and intubated, physical findings may be blunted.

Laboratory findings that tend to be significant include a leukocytosis with left shift and elevated alkaline phosphatase. Ultrasonographically, although there is an absence of gallstones, findings that may suggest acalculous cholecystitis include gallbladder distention, wall thickening, and sludge within the lumen. These findings, however, may also be seen in the sick intensive care unit patient without acalculous cholecystitis. If further evidence of disease is still required, a HIDA scan can be performed. The accuracy in this setting is less than that in acute cholecystitis, since most of these patients have not had oral intake for prolonged periods. Failure to visualize the gallbladder does not confirm the diagnosis, but visualization of the gallbladder effectively rules out acalculous cholecystitis.

TABLE 8. DIFFERENTIATION OF ACUTE VERSUS CHRONIC CHOLECYSTITIS

	History	Pain Pattern*	Pain Location	Associated Findings	Temperature	Laboratory
Acute Cholecystitis	Acute onset of pain, usually following a fatty meal	Constant, moderately severe pain lasting typically >6h; often unrelieved by narcotics	Epigastrium to RUQ. Localizes in RUQ to right mid-abdomen (hydrops). Gallbladder may be palpable. Murphy's sign strongly +.	Nausea, vomiting frequent	Elevated (may only be 99°–100° F)	WBC ↑ (10 000–15 000) LFTs typically normal, although alkaline phosphatase, t. bili, and transaminases may be mildly ↑
Chronic cholecystitis	Acute onset of pain, usually following a fatty meal	Constant, moderately severe pain, but typically lasting <6h and often relieved by narcotics	Epigastrium to RUQ, not well localized. Murphy's sign − or equivocal.	Nausea, vomiting variable	Normal	WBC normal, alkaline phosphatase, t. bili, and transaminases may be mildly ↑ if patient passed a stone, otherwise LFTs are normal

* Most important differentiating point

LFT, liver function tests; RUQ, right upper quadrant; WBC, white blood cell.

Biliary Dyskinesia

On occasion, a patient will describe a "classic" episode of pain of presumed biliary tract origin. This episode of RUQ pain typically follows a fatty meal and radiates around the back to the scapula. There may be associated nausea and vomiting. Laboratory data are normal. Much to everyone's surprise, however, the ultrasonogram reveals no gallstones. The diagnostic exploration may be extensive in search of other pathologic conditions. It may include exclusion of peptic and gastric ulcers, computed tomographic (CT) scans of the abdomen, ERCP, and even produce a label of psychosis. In this subgroup of patients, a diagnosis of biliary dyskinesia should be entertained. It is believed that in the patients who suffer from this problem, the gallbladder fails to effectively contract and empty in response to CCK. Normally, the gallbladder will empty about 50% of its bile in response to a physiologic dose of CCK. This ejection fraction can be quantified with the use of the radionuclide scan. Patients with "classic" biliary symptoms, negative ultrasonograms, and less than a 50% ejection fraction on HIDA scan after the slow injection of a CCK analog have been shown to respond favorably to cholecystectomy.

Choledocholithiasis

The presence of stones within the common bile duct is termed choledocholithiasis. These stones may originate within the gallbladder and pass into the common bile duct or form de novo within the duct even after previous cholecystectomy. Choledocholithiasis exists in two forms, symptomatic and asymptomatic. Symptomatic stones can serve as a nidus of obstruction within the biliary tree and present with four possible manifestations, depending on the extent as well as level of obstruction: biliary colic, jaundice, cholangitis, or pancreatitis. Asymptomatic stones are usually identified with cholangiography in as many as 15% of patients undergoing cholecystectomy.

Obstruction initiates a chain of events, starting with an increase of intraductal pressure. At times this increase in intraductal pressure may be sufficient to promote spontaneous passage of the lodged stone. If this does not occur, proximal ductal dilatation and complications may occur.

The pain associated with choledocholithiasis is similar to that of cholecystitis, a deep-seated visceral pain with only minor fluctuations in intensity. Usually it is midepigastric or in the RUQ, with radiation to the back. The pain may be girdlelike if the stone is impacted at the level of the ampulla of Vater. Jaundiced patients may notice darkening of their urine or light or acholic stools with chronic obstruction. Nausea and vomiting may be among the signs and symptoms. The patient commonly complains of back pain. Laboratory findings may be normal in the asymptomatic group, although unsuspected elevations in alkaline phosphatase or bilirubin may be noted on screening liver function tests. When symptomatic, patients may have clinical and biochemical jaundice, elevated alkaline phosphatase, and elevated transaminases. An elevated alkaline phosphatase alone is not a very sensitive indicator of choledocholithiasis, but when combined with ductal dilatation or elevated bilirubin, the sensitivity of this biliary canalicular enzyme is enhanced.

In addition, the level of elevation does not correlate with the degree of obstruction. Bilirubin elevation is typically noted after abnormalities of alkaline phosphatase. Peak levels are generally 2 to 10mg/dL with higher levels noted in hepatic parenchymal disease or malignant obstruction. Fluctuating jaundice is so characteristic of choledocholithiasis that it helps differentiate between benign and malignant obstruction.

Diagnostic procedures to evaluate choledocholithiasis include ultrasonography, ERCP, PTC, and HIDA. Ultrasonography can demonstrate either the stone within the CBD (rarely) or ductal dilatation (more commonly). More accurate information regarding the presence of choledocholithiasis can be obtained with ERCP or PTC. If a HIDA scan is performed in the presence of complete CBD obstruction, radionuclide will fail to visualize the duodenum.

Cholangitis

Obstruction of the extrahepatic bile ducts, regardless of the origin, can lead to cholangitis. Bacterial presence in the biliary tree in the absence of obstruction does not produce symptoms or pathologic changes. Obstruction to bile flow produces an increase in ductal pressure and subsequent retrograde ductal dilatation. The combination of bacteribilia and biliary stasis or obstruction leads to cholangitis. The principle causes of biliary obstruction include choledocholithiasis, biliary stricture, or neoplasm.

The pathophysiology of cholangitis explains the common presentation: fever with chills (secondary to bacteremia), RUQ pain, and jaundice. Collectively, these three symptoms are known as Charcot's triad. Laboratory tests of significance may include a leukocytosis of 15 000 to 20 000 with a left shift. Blood cultures may be positive in 50% of patients. Elevation of the alkaline phosphatase and transaminases are also seen.

A more virulent form of cholangitis is found in 15% of patients and is termed toxic or suppurative cholangitis. In toxic cholangitis the obstruction to the biliary tree is usually more complete, as compared to conventional cholangitis, and this leads to purulent bile under pressure within the biliary system. It is this pathophysiologic sequence that leads to bacteremia and sepsis. It is the combination of Charcot's triad with hypotension and mental status changes associated with sepsis that produce Reynold's pentad of suppurative cholangitis.

THE DIFFERENTIAL DIAGNOSIS OF RUQ PAIN

Pleuritis or Right-sided Pneumonia

A right-sided basilar pneumonia or pleurisy may present with acute abdominal findings. The patient may complain of pain in the RUQ of the abdomen with a corresponding area of tenderness. In contrast to acute cholecystitis, the pain of pleurisy or pneumonia tends to be exacerbated with a deep inspiratory effort. A history of productive sputum or cough also suggests an intrathoracic process as the source of the RUQ pain. Physical examination may disclose a high fever (102° to 104° F), which is atypical for uncomplicated cholecystitis and more compatible with pneumonia. Auscultation of the lung fields may reveal a rub, and consolidation may be demonstrable with diminished breath sounds. The abdominal tenderness that may be present with pleurisy or pneumonia is superficial compared with the tenderness of cholecystitis, which is much deeper. As always, a chest roentgenogram should be ordered for anyone with abdominal pain and should clarify any confusion.

Hepatitis

Alcoholic hepatitis may have an abrupt onset or exacerbation, presenting with RUQ pain and tenderness as well as a low-grade fever. In alcoholic hepatitis, mild elevations in both the WBC count and liver function tests only add further confusion in differentiating this process from acute cholecystitis. In hepatitis, the acute swelling of Glisson's capsule of the liver is the mechanism of RUQ pain. Unlike cholecystitis in which the tenderness is overlying the gallbladder, in hepatitis the entire liver is tender. Thus palpation of the lateral aspect of the liver in the midaxillary line will reproduce the pain in hepatitis but not in cholecystitis. Women presenting with RUQ abdominal pain and tenderness with associated cervical and adnexal tenderness should be suspected of having gonococcal perihepatitis (Fitz–Hugh–Curtis syndrome). Auscultation in the RUQ may reveal a friction rub resulting from the numerous adhesions that form between the abdominal wall and the liver.

Renal Disease

Pain in the anterior abdominal wall may be induced by the passage of renal calculi. The pain will radiate from the flank to the groin. A history of dysuria may be reported. Physical examination of the abdomen may reveal some voluntary guarding and signs consistent with an ileus. Costovertebral angle tenderness may be elicited on the affected side. Examination of the urine for the presence of either hematuria, crystals, renal casts, or bacteria aids in the diagnosis.

Acute Appendicitis

Most instances of acute appendicitis can be ascertained on the basis of a compatible history and physical examination (see Chapter 5). However, a long, retrocecal, acutely inflamed appendix may present with RUQ pain. In general, appendicitis progresses more rapidly, over 12 to 24 hours, compared to cholecystitis, which may smolder for days. To add more confusion to the situation, a hydrops of the gallbladder may present with more right lower quadrant (RLQ) and right midabdominal pain, although in the latter condition the gallbladder is usually palpable. A low-lying hydropic gallbladder and a long, retrocecal appendix may be difficult to distinguish between clinically; even a good diagnostician occasionally makes an ill-placed incision during the course of his or her career.

Peptic Ulcer Disease

Anatomically, the gallbladder and duodenum are in close proximity. Therefore, diseases of one organ may mimic symptoms of the other. A past history of peptic ulcer disease may help in the differential diagnosis, and therefore this information should be sought in the interview. The symptom of dyspepsia associated with chronic cholecystitis may mimic the symptoms of ulcer disease. In addition, the patient with a duodenal ulcer may also have cholelithiasis, thereby making the differentiation between the two difficult. In general, the pain of an ulcer is relieved with a meal, whereas the opposite is true of cholecystitis. Antacids, commonly consumed by the patient for complaints of abdominal pain, should improve ulcers and be ineffectual for cholecystitis. When the symptoms are not typical of cholecystitis, it is a reasonable approach to exclude an ulcer with either an esophagogastroduodenoscopy or a contrast study. A perforated ulcer is usually much easier to differentiate from acute cholecystitis on the basis of the history, a thorough abdominal examination, and free air noted on abdominal radiographs.

Acute Pancreatitis

Alcohol, gallstones, and drugs remain the prevalent causes of acute pancreatitis. Therefore, assuming gallstones are not the issue, a history of alcohol ingestion or medication usage should be obtainable by history or from the family. Thiazide diuretics, steroids, or azathioprine are the predominate medications known to incite pancreatitis. In acute pancreatitis, the pain tends to be more severe with more associated nausea, vomiting, and wretching. While the pain of cholecystitis may be noted in the epigastrium, it ultimately localizes to the RUQ and commonly radiates around to the back. Pancreatitis, however, tends to have its maximal pain located in the epigastrium. More commonly, the pain of pancreatitis radiates to the left side and straight through to the back rather than around the sides. Patients with pancreatitis look sicker than patients with cholecystitis. Amylase and lipase levels, while not specific for pancreatitis, are usually elevated with pancreatic inflammation and are not in uncomplicated acute cholecystitis. The exception is gallstone pancreatitis. It is reasonable to exclude gallstones in any patient presenting with clinical and laboratory evidence of pancreatitis.

Herpes Zoster

Herpes zoster, also called shingles, is an acute eruption of the latent herpes virus within a nerve ganglion and its overlying areas of cutaneous innervation. The pain associated with herpes zoster is characteristically burning or stabbing in nature. If the involved ganglia innervated the RUQ of the abdomen, it can be confused with acute cholecystitis. In shingles, an erythematous maculopapular rash lies over the involved dermatome, although its clinical appearance may lag behind the onset of the pain, adding further confusion to the diagnosis.

Myocardial Ischemia or Infarction
An acute inferior wall myocardial infarction or accelerating angina may produce intense epigastric abdominal pain. Nausea and vomiting may also be noted and add to the confusion with cholecystitis. Objective abdominal examination is usually normal, although occasionally the patient may have voluntary guarding in the epigastric region. If the onset of pain occurred during the ingestion of a meal, the diagnosis may be even more confused with biliary tract disease. The key to the diagnosis of myocardial ischemia rests upon a thorough history, enumeration of risk factors, and the electrocardiogram and appropriate cardiac enzyme analysis. If cholecystitis is suspected and the ultrasonogram shows no stones, a cardiac source for the pain should be considered. The more difficult situation is that of the patient with cholelithiasis, no evidence of acute cholecystitis, and the examiner's concern about overlooking cardiac disease. The examiner must always maintain a high index of suspicion for occult cardiac disease, especially in the high-risk individual.

SUGGESTED READING

Brooks, JR. Acute and chronic cholecystitis. In: Cameron JL, ed. *Current Surgical Therapy.* 3rd ed. Toronto, Ont: BC Decker Inc; 1989.

Davis GB, Berk RN, Sheible FW, et al. Cholecystokinin cholecystography, sonography and scintigraphy: detection of chronic acalculous cholecystitis. *AJR Am J Roentgenal.* 1982; 139:1117–1121.

DenBesten L, Roslyn JJ. Gallstones and cholecystitis. In: Moody F, et al, eds. *Surgical Treatment of Digestive Disease.* Chicago, Ill: Year Book Medical Publishers Inc; 1986.

Kune Ga, Gill GD. Cholecystitis. In: Schwartz SI, Ellis H, eds. *Maingot's Abdominal Operations.* 9th ed. Norwalk, Conn: Appleton and Lange; 1990.

McSherry CK, et al. The natural history of diagnosed gallstone disease in symptomatic and asymptomatic patients. *Ann Surg.* 1985; 202:59.

Schoenfield LJ. Gallstones. *Clin Symp.* 1988; 40:2.

Sharp KW. Acute cholecystitis. *Surg Clin North Am.* 1988; 68:269.

Way LW, Sleisenger MH. Acute cholecystitis. In: Sleisenger MH, Fordtran JS, eds. *Gastrointestinal Disease: Pathology Diagnosis, Management.* 3rd ed. Philadelphia, Pa: WB Saunders Co; 1983.

Welch JP. Intestinal obstruction. In: Welch JP, ed. *Bowel Obstruction: Differential Diagnosis and Clinical Management.* Philadelphia, Pa: WB Saunders Co; 1990.

CHAPTER 7

■

Pancreatitis

Joseph M. Vitello, MD
Bernardo Duarte, MD

ACUTE PANCREATITIS

Acute pancreatitis is a disease with a wide spectrum of manifestations. A mild attack may present with little abdominal pain and resolve in a day or two. A fulminant attack may be complicated by hypovolemic shock, multiple-system organ failure, and death. Between these two extremes a variable course may exist. Chronic pancreatitis also produces abdominal pain and should be considered in the differential diagnosis of any patient with upper abdominal complaints, especially those patients with previous attacks of acute pancreatitis.

Pancreatitis should always be considered in the assessment of patients with acute abdominal pain, especially those patients known to consume alcohol, to have gallstones or who have had a recent diagnostic procedure, eg, endoscopic retrograde cholangiopancreatography, either with or without papillotomy. Recent surgery, abdominal trauma, and certain drugs are other risk factors that may predispose a patient to the development of pancreatitis. A list of factors known to induce pancreatitis is reproduced in Table 9. Despite this lengthy list of known precipitating factors, approximately 10% of pancreatitis instances will have no identifiable cause. Any patient with persistent epigastric pain of more than 24 to 48 hours' duration who does not obtain relief with common analgesics should be suspected of having pancreatitis.

The pathophysiology of acute pancreatitis appears to be the liberation and activation of pancreatic proteolytic enzymes, with autodigestion and destruction of the gland and surrounding tissues. Activated enzymes such as trypsin, chymotrypsin, elastase, and phospholipase A cause digestion of cellular membranes leading to proteolysis, edema, interstitial hemorrhage, vas-

119

TABLE 9. COMMON CAUSES OF ACUTE PANCREATITIS

1. Alcohol consumption
2. Gallstones
3. Trauma
   blunt abdominal
   penetrating abdominal
4. Postoperative causes
   abdominal surgery, especially upper abdominal
   extra-abdominal surgery
5. Postprocedural causes
   ERCP
   sphincterotomy
   cardiopulmonary bypass
6. Drug-induced causes
   thiazide diuretics
   corticosteroids
   azathioprine
   sulfonamides
   furosemide
   estrogens
   tetracycline
7. Peptic ulcer disease
8. Metabolic causes
   hyperlipidemia (especially types I and V)
   hypercalcemia
   hypotensive shock
9. Hereditary pancreatitis
10. Infections
    mumps
    other viral illnesses (coxsackie)
    ascariasis
    mycoplasma
    legionnaires' disease
    tuberculosis
11. Connective tissue diseases
    systemic lupus erythematosus
    polyarteritis nodosum
12. Pancreas divisum
13. Scorpion bites
14. Pancreatic cancer
15. Choledochal cyst
16. Cystic fibrosis
17. Idiopathic causes

cular damage, coagulation, and fat necrosis, and cellular death. Pancreatitis is a disease with local, regional, and systemic effects of varying severity.

It is essential to remember the anatomy of the pancreas and its relationship to neighboring structures. The location is in the retroperitoneum, and it is intimately related to the common bile duct and duodenum. Furthermore, its position also relates to the stomach, proximal jejunum, and transverse colon, kidneys, and spleen. Most importantly, the retroperitoneal position of the pancreas allows an inflammatory process access into the mediastinum and thorax, root of the small-intestinal mesentary, the paracolic gutters, and even down into the scrotum or femoral canals. The acute pancreatic process may, according to its magnitude and severity, affect any of the neighboring organs. A single organ may be involved, or a combination of them. The entire process may not remain confined to the retroperitoneum, but necessitate or rupture free into the coelom and present as any kind of an acute abdomen with peritonitis. The pancreas has sympathetic innervation from the splanchnic nerves, which coalesce in the celiac plexus. The pancreas lies directly over this plexus, which explains the mechanism of pain transmission and the degree of back discomfort associated with pancreatic inflammation. As with any complaint of abdominal pain, the historical account of the problem may aid in the determination of the exact diagnosis. With pancreatitis, known precipitating events or drugs should be thoroughly explored in the history. In general, pancreatitis is uncommon in children. Alcoholic and traumatic pancreatitis tends to be more common in men, whereas gallstone pancreatitis is seen more frequently in women. Oftentimes, pancreatitis is a recurring problem, and this should be ascertained in the history. It must be remembered that the diagnosis of acute or chronic pancreatitis is one of exclusion. Failure to consider pancreatitis in the differential diagnosis of the patient's abdominal pain is one of the chief reasons the diagnosis is missed. A potential problem is that upon presentation, many common clinical conditions mimic pancreatitis, eg, perforated duodenal ulcer or acute cholecystitis. Alternatively, pancreatitis may mimic other forms of acute abdomen, such as intestinal obstruction, perforated viscus, or ischemic bowel. These facts make the history of the affected patient extremely important. Failure to detect underlying alcoholism may not only obscure the diagnosis of pancreatitis but leads to neglect of treatment for the primary disorder. The background information of known cholelithiasis, recent trauma, or drug therapy are also important points that should not be omitted from the history.

Onset

The most common presenting symptom of pancreatitis is abdominal pain, which may vary in intensity or severity. The majority of attacks follow overindulgence in food or alcohol. The pain may start at any time of day or night. The pain usually begins insidiously, but episodes of severe, acute pain with pallor and diaphoresis may be found in patients who present in shock.

The attack usually persists for more than 36 to 48 hours, with no relief before presentation at the hospital. The pain is usually located in the epigastrium, with radiation to both sides of the upper abdomen and to the back, but not usually to the tip of the scapula as is typical of acute cholecystitis. Instead, the back pain is lower, usually between the kidneys. Classically, the pain is described as piercing from front to back, as though the patient had been shot with an arrow in the epigastrium. The anatomic position of the gland logically explains the location of the pain.

The Physical Findings

The patient's position and facial expression may give an indication as to the severity of the disease. Typically, in acute pancreatitis the patient looks sick. Lying on his or her side in the fetal or knee-to-chest position offers symptomatic relief by "relaxing" the pancreas. Although patients often assume this position, it is not ordinarily helpful and therefore they tend to periodically shift themselves in an attempt to alleviate the pain. Typically, narcotics are required to relieve the pain of acute pancreatitis. The physical findings are dependent on the severity of the attack, the duration of the process, and the timing of presentation. The physician may be impressed by a confused, indifferent, languid individual. The patient may be moribund and in shock if presented late in the disease process. The majority of patients present with signs of hypovolemia, diaphoresis, and hypotension, or slightly flushed with tachycardia and mild hypertension. The different presentations are manifestations of the systemic effect of cytokines and other inflammatory mediators released during pancreatitis.

Tachycardia is usually evident and is a result of pain and hypovolemia. In severe acute pancreatitis with associated pancreatic necrosis or hemorrhage, shock may result. The definition of shock is inadequate tissue perfusion and not necessarily the presence of unstable vital signs. Hypovolemic shock develops as a result of the tremendous amount of fluid that may be sequestered in the retroperitoneum and the surrounding structures. As the disease progresses, however, shock may be secondary to any one of several complications, such as rupture of a pseudocyst or sepsis. Regardless of the exact cause, shock creates a set of physiologic responses producing distinctive physical findings. Cool, clammy skin is not specific for pancreatitis but merely reflects a physiologic response to shock. When shock occurs in association with pancreatitis it is an ominous sign, with significant mortality.

Temperature. Fever is not usually higher than one or two degrees above normal. Fever may progress and become significantly elevated, even in the absence of definite infection. This is probably related to the severity of pancreatic inflammation and peripancreatic necrosis and is caused by cytokine release.

Respiratory Compromise. Tachypnea, dyspnea, and subtle hypoxia are commonly observed during an attack of acute pancreatitis. This is partially due to anxiety and pain. In addition, pleural effusions and hydrothorax occur frequently. The pleural effusion is preferentially on the left side and usually occurs early in the disease process. This results in pleuritis. Other subdiaphragmatic entities like acute cholecystitis or perforated ulcer may lead to diaphragmatic splinting, but this is less common with pancreatitis. Abdominal distention may also contribute to respiratory compromise and lead to dyspnea. While respiratory distress in acute pancreatitis may be due to atelectasis, interstitial edema, or pneumonia, the most catastrophic event is the development of adult respiratory distress syndrome (ARDS). Respiratory failure may develop suddenly, with disastrous consequences. Therefore, arterial blood gas determination should be performed early in the assessment of anyone suspected of having acute pancreatitis.

Jaundice. Jaundice may be encountered in some cases and is indicative of swelling of the head of the pancreas with impingement on the distal common bile duct or an impacted gallstone at the ampulla of Vater. When this occurs, scleral icterus is easily identifiable.

Vomiting. Vomiting is the second most frequent symptom in pancreatitis and in most circumstances is preceded by pain. Vomiting does not result in relief of symptoms as it does with some abdominal problems; instead repeated vomiting and retching only serves to worsen the pain. Reflex vomiting commonly persists even after the stomach has been emptied. This persistent retching with nonproductive vomiting is somewhat characteristic of pancreatitis. In acute pancreatitis, vomiting may be massive, with severe electrolyte imbalance and significant fluid losses. The character of the vomitus is bilious, since it usually contains gastric and duodenal fluids. The presence of blood is rare and, when it occurs, should be thought of as a complication of the disease.

Gastrointestinal Effects. Diarrhea and gastrointestinal bleeding may be found in extensive hemorrhagic pancreatitis; therefore the patient may present with hematemesis or melena.

Inspection of the Abdomen. Visual inspection of the abdominal contour may reveal distention. Since an ileus commonly accompanies an attack of pancreatitis, this explains the degree of distention. However, other causes such as ascites and hemoperitoneum should always be kept in the differential diagnosis. The often quoted Cullen's sign (periumbilical ecchymosis) and Grey Turner's sign (flank ecchymosis) are not commonly seen and, when noted, occur late in the disease. Furthermore, these signs are not specific for pancreatitis but merely reflect the presence of retroperitoneal blood.

Auscultation of the Abdomen. The ileus in acute pancreatitis may be minor at the early stages, with preservation of bowel sounds. When the pancreatitis is progressive and severe, the ileus becomes generalized and involves the stomach, duodenum, proximal small intestine, and colon. Therefore, in the late stages of the disease, the ileus may be a significant feature in the clinical presentation, leading to a different diagnosis, such as intestinal obstruction or ischemic bowel.

Percussion and Palpation of the Abdomen

At the onset of acute pancreatitis there may be a disparity between the severity of symptoms and the paucity of physical findings. Percussion may aid in the delineation of abdominal fluid, liver span, or outline a pseudocyst. Early in pancreatitis, there may be mild abdominal pain with some localized guarding. Initially, tenderness and guarding exist in the epigastrium and upper quadrants. Maximal tenderness tends to remain in the midline but as the disease progresses, the examination may reveal a more generalized peritonitis suggestive of a perforated ulcer. Rebound tenderness and rigidity may become the predominant finding but do not necessarily signify an immediate surgical problem. However, when peritoneal findings are observed, secondary complication may occur and need to be excluded. Examples include necrosis of the greater curvature of the stomach or transverse colon, or the development of an abscess, all of which obviously require surgical intervention. For these reasons the diagnosis of pancreatitis can be extremely challenging.

Palpation may also reveal a mass if a phlegmon or pseudocyst is developing. This mass is usually noted just below the xiphoid and costal margins and is commonly tender to palpation, with associated guarding.

Central Nervous System. Occasionally, pancreatitis may be complicated by the development of delirium tremens, which worsens and complicates the overall situation. Since many patients with pancreatitis also abuse alcohol, delirium tremens should be anticipated and treated. Thiamine should be administered prophylactically to prevent Wernicke's encephalopathy.

Laboratory Evaluation

The white blood cell count is typically elevated in the range of 15 000 to 20 000. In instances of severe pancreatitis, especially complicated by abscess, the white count can easily be seen to reach 30 000 to 50 000. The hematocrit tends to be elevated because of hemoconcentration, although it may fall when hemorrhage is a component of the pancreatitis. Hyperglycemia is commonly noted. This occurs both because of the stress response and because many of these patients have a history of recurrent pancreatitis and have developed endocrine insufficiency.

The interpretation of an isolated laboratory value of hyperamylasemia as diagnostic of acute pancreatitis can prove erroneous, since many pathologic conditions can result in amylase elevation (Table 10). An appropriate history combined with an elevated amylase level is, however, highly suggestive of pancreatitis. Serum amylase is typically elevated in acute pancreatitis; however, the severity of the disease does not correlate with the degree of amylase elevation. Amylase is cleared rapidly in the urine. The clearance of amylase exceeds that of creatinine, so that in the patient presenting late in the disease, the serum amylase may actually be normal or normalizing. For that reason

TABLE 10. CAUSES OF HYPERAMYLASEMIA

1. Pancreatic disease
   acute pancreatitis and its complications
   chronic pancreatitis and its complications
   carcinoma of the pancreas
   pancreatic trauma
2. Nonpancreatic disease
   renal insufficiency
   salivary gland pathology
      mumps
      calculus
      irradiation sialadenitis
      maxillofacial surgery
3. Macroamylasemia
4. Intra-abdominal disease other than pancreatic in origin
   perforated peptic ulcer
   intestinal obstruction
   ruptured ectopic pregnancy
   acute salpingitis
   ovarian torsion
   intestinal infarction
   afferent loop syndrome
   ruptured aortic aneurysm or dissection
   peritonitis
   acute appendicitis
   acute cholecystitis
   perforated diverticulitis
5. Cerebral trauma
6. Burns and traumatic shock
7. Diabetic ketoacidosis
8. Renal transplantation
9. Pneumonia
10. Prostatic disease
11. Pregnancy
12. Drugs

there are those who advocate use of the urine amylase:creatinine ratio. This laboratory assessment has been found to be nonspecific, however.

Two isoenzymes of amylase exist: p, or pancreatic and s, or salivary. Most circulating amylase is normally salivary. However, in pancreatitis, the p-amylase accounts for about 75% of total amylase in more than 50% of patients. The clinical usefulness of amylase isoenzyme determination is yet to be fully elucidated. Lipase levels tend to rise in parallel with amylase, but their levels fall more slowly. For this reason, this enzyme may be more useful in those patients who present later in the course of their disease, after serum amylase levels have already normalized.

Elevated triglyceride levels are commonly observed. Hyperlipidemia can be both cause and effect in pancreatitis; therefore an assessment for one of the congenital hyperlipidemias seems appropriate if triglycerides are outside the normal range.

Calcium levels may fall as a result of the sequestration of this divalent ion in the saponification process and precipitation of calcium soaps within the abdominal cavity. Since the fall in calcium may be precipitous and result in tetany, it should be followed closely. With the development of the ionized calcium electrode, this component of total serum calcium is more appropriately monitored.

Because the course of pancreatitis varies, on admission to the hospital it is difficult to determine the severity of a given case. For this reason, prognostic variables have been outlined by Ranson. These criteria predict the mortality of acute pancreatitis. The tests in and of themselves are not diagnostic of pancreatitis but are listed so that the physician can be aware to order the appropriate tests in a predictive fashion. (Table 11).

Radiology

Abdominal radiographs may reveal distended gas-filled loops of both small and large intestine, a pattern distinctive for an ileus. Occasionally, an isolated loop of distended small bowel appears in the upper abdomen. This so called sentinel loop is not specific for pancreatitis but reflects an inflammatory focus irritating a segment of intestine. If the ileus affects the transverse colon, there may be air up to that point, with a paucity of distal colonic air. This is referred to as a colon cut-off sign and mimics an obstructing carcinoma. Calcifications along the length of the pancreas noted on plain abdominal roentgenograms suggest frequent recurrent attacks of pancreatitis. In addition, plain abdominal radiographs may demonstrate gallstones. Chest radiographs may disclose a pleural effusion or free air leading to an alternate diagnosis.

Barium upper gastrointestinal examinations are of historic interest in the diagnosis of acute pancreatitis. Ultrasonography is useful to define gallstones and pseudocysts but often cannot completely survey the pancreas because of the severity of the ileus. The best study to evaluate the pancreas is computed

TABLE 11. RANSON'S CRITERIA FOR ACUTE PANCREATITIS

On Admission

Age > 55
WBC > 16 000
Glucose > 200mg/dL
LDH > 350 U/L
AST (SGOT) > 250 U/L

After 48 Hours

Hematocrit drop > 10%
BUN increase > 5mg/dL
Calcium < 8.0
pO < 60mm Hg on room air
Base deficit > 4mEq/L
Estimated fluid sequestration > 6 L

Number of Signs	*Mortality*
3–4	20%
5–6	40%
>6	100%

AST (SGOT), aspartate transaminate (serum glutamic-oxalo-acetic transaminase), BUN, blood urea nitrogen; LDH, lactate dehydrogenase; WBC, white blood cell.

tomography (CT). This study, unaffected by overlying bowel gas, not only outlines the pancreas but also delineates the degree of peripancreatic inflammation.

Complications of Acute Pancreatitis

Pseudocyst formation is a common complication of acute pancreatitis. Typically, a patient who is recovering nicely from an episode of pancreatitis develops a persistently palpable mass, pain, or elevated amylase level. A pancreatic pseudocyst may develop in or from the head, body, or tail of the gland. The pseudocyst wall is actually composed of the surrounding inflammatory tissue and organs and contains no epithelial lining, hence the name pseudocyst. The cyst often contains blood, pancreatic enzymes, and necrotic debris. The natural history of the pseudocyst varies. Smaller pseudocysts may resolve spontaneously. Large cysts (>5cm), which often produce pain, typically require intervention. Other complications of the pseudocyst include infection, erosion into nearby organs, free rupture into the peritoneal cavity with the development of pancreatic ascites, or hemorrhage caused by erosion into nearby vascular structures. If the pseudocyst is located in the head of the pancreas, nausea, vomiting, and early satiety occur as a result of gastric outlet obstruction, pylorospasm, or delayed gastric emptying. Diagnosis can be suspected on physical examination by the detection of a palpable mass in a patient with resolving pancreatitis. Ultrasound and CT confirm the clinical impression and define the extent.

Infectious Complications. Infectious complications can occur after an attack of acute pancreatitis. Whether this takes the form of an abscess or infected pancreatic necrosis, the result is the same. Operative drainage and debridement are essential. The mechanism of bacterial infection is a subject of some debate. Infected bile or hematogenous seeding have been postulated. The most common organisms are coliforms, which leads to the suspicion that transmigration of intestinal organisms represents the actual mechanism. The extent of infection may be confined to a pseudocyst, the pancreatic tissue, or extend to any area that has been affected by the inflammatory process, ie, retroperitoneum, pelvis, small-intestinal mesentery, or paracolonic gutters. Typically these patients are very ill, with persistently high fevers, chills, positive blood cultures, and impressive leukocystosis. Drainage is essential; inadequate drainage can result in death.

Hemorrhagic Complications. Massive hemorrhage associated with pancreatitis is rare but often fatal when it occurs. There may be bleeding into the intestinal tract, the retroperitoneum, or the peritoneal cavity. The bleeding may be due to liquifaction necrosis of peripancreatic vessels or erosion into major arteries such as the splenic artery.

Differential Diagnosis

Perforated Ulcer. Acute perforation of an ulcer may be confused with pancreatitis. To help distinguish the two, known history of an ulcer should be elicited. With ulcer perforation, the onset of pain is acute and reaches its maximum intensity at once, with associated rigidity. The abdomen is usually more diffusely tender and rigid early in the course of symptoms, whereas pancreatitis progresses more insidiously. Abdominal radiographs usually demonstrate free air. Serum amylase levels may be elevated in either situation and thus do not suggest one diagnosis over the other.

Appendicitis. The prodromes are more gradual with appendicitis than with pancreatitis, and the severity of pain and vomiting are less. Patients with pancreatitis appear sicker. Ultimately, when pain localizes in the right lower quadrant, epigastric tenderness has abated and pancreatitis is removed from the differential diagnosis.

Intestinal Obstruction. Intestinal obstruction is suspected when abdominal pain occurs in a patient with previous abdominal surgery and with obstipation. The pain of intestinal obstruction is crampy, whereas in pancreatitis it is constant. If abdominal distention is present, the two entities can be difficult to distinguish, since a severe ileus associated with pancreatitis can mimic intestinal obstruction. Bowel sounds associated with intestinal obstruction tend to be hyperactive, with borborygmi, whereas with pancreatitis, the activity is minimal. Once again, amylase levels may be elevated in either condition.

Acute Cholecystitis or Biliary Colic. With biliary tract disease the pain is located more in the right upper quadrant and is less severe than with pancreatitis. Although nausea and vomiting may be prominent in biliary tract disease, they tend to resolve early. Symptomatic improvement may be attained in the patient with biliary tract disease by allowing nothing by mouth and starting intravenous fluid. A dose of narcotic usually improves the pain of cholecystitis. These measures often do not help the patient with pancreatitis.

Mesenteric Vascular Occlusion. Pain onset with this disease is slow and progressive. The pain is typically out of proportion to the physical finding, with the patient writhing. Risk factors for embolic mesenteric ischemia include atrial fibrillation, recent myocardial infarction, or known peripheral vascular disease. Ultimately blood is passed in the stool, which is uncommon with pancreatitis. Once again, amylase elevation is commonly seen in both of these entities.

Myocardial Infarction. The pain is typically crushing and substernal, often radiating to the jaw or arm. Objective abdominal findings are minimal. The electrocardiogram and elevations of cardiac enzymes secure the diagnosis.

CHRONIC PANCREATITIS

Chronic pancreatitis occurs in patients who have had recurrent episodes of acute pancreatitis, most commonly from alcoholism. Chronic pancreatitis typically presents as an acute attack and has been referred to as chronic relapsing pancreatitis.

A persistent form of chronic pancreatitis without acute exacerbations is characterized by constant abdominal and back pain, worsened by food ingestion. Commonly these patients have developed exocrine and endocrine pancreatic insufficiency. Obstruction of the main pancreatic duct and its tributaries with calculi results in pain. The calcifications can commonly be seen on plain abdominal radiographs. They represent the precipitation of amorphous protein in the ducts, which calcifies and creates surrounding inflammation and obstruction. The obstruction creates cystic dilatation within the main pancreatic duct. This process occurs repeatedly along the main duct until a "chain of lakes" is formed representing intermittent constriction and dilated cystic components of the main duct.

Pain is the most common and important clinical symptom in these patients. The pain tends to be constant and exacerbated by eating. The location of the pain is typically in the epigastrium, with a large component of back discomfort. Radiation to the upper quadrants is less common with chronic pancreatitis but may be present. Because of the exacerbated pain on eating, patients commonly avoid food, lose weight, and become malnourished. For this reason these patients look chronically ill. The patients typically require narcotics for the relief of their pain. Not uncommonly the patient has seen several physicians and visited many emergency rooms. Repeated issuance of prescriptions for narcotics often leads to iatrogenic drug dependence. Persistent alcohol consumption serves to exacerbate the whole process. As ongoing destruction of the gland occurs, the patients develop exocrine insufficiency, which leads to fat malabsorption and steatorrhea. In addition, endocrine dysfunction develops, leading to diabetes. This inexorable course of calcifications, diabetes, and steatorrhea, which occurs over the course of 15 to 20 years, leads ultimately to death.

GALLSTONE PANCREATITIS

The common channel theory has been invoked to account for the occurrence of gallstone pancreatitis. A gallstone migrating down the common bile duct is believed to pass the opening of the main pancreatic duct and produce pancreatitis. The stones could be recovered in the stool if one were to search. While some of these patients develop full-blown pancreatitis, others are noted to have transient pain and a markedly elevated amylase (>2000 IU). Within 24 hours symptoms resolve and amylase levels fall precipitously. Although the amylase elevations are striking, the clinical course appears benign, reaffirming that the amylase level does not correlate with the severity of pancreatitis. Once ultrasonography confirms cholelithiasis, a timely cholecystectomy should be performed.

CONCLUSION

Pancreatitis in either its acute or chronic form, regardless of underlying etiology, may present a variable course. A thorough history and a high degree of suspicion lead to the diagnosis. Epigastric pain predominates among the clinical signs and symptoms. Elevation of amylase levels, while not specific, is supportive for the diagnosis. Procurement of the appropriate laboratory studies may be helpful in predicting the course and severity of disease in individuals presenting with acute pancreatitis. CT is probably the imaging study of choice to detect the extent of pancreatitis and to screen for many of the complications of this challenging disease.

SUGGESTED READING

Burns GP, Bank S. *Disorders of the Pancreas: Current Issues in Diagnosis and Management.* New York, NY: McGraw-Hill Book Co Inc; 1992.

Laycock R, Pemberton LB, Coffey RR, et al. Pancreas. In: Lawrence, ed. *Essentials of Surgery.* 2nd ed. Baltimore, Md: Williams & Wilkins; 1992.

Salt WB, Schenker S. Amylase—its clinical significance: a review of the literature. *Medicine.* 1976; 55:269–289.

CHAPTER 8

■

Diverticulitis

Colanthur Palani, MD

The incidence of diverticula of the colon increases with advancing age and adoption of diet low in fiber content. Diverticula are produced when increased pressure in the lumen of the colon forces the mucosal layer through weakness in the muscular wall at blood vessel entry sites. These diverticula lack the muscular layer and thus are pseudodiverticula, as opposed to true diverticula, which have all the three layers of the intestine. Diverticulitis, a serious complication of colonic diverticulosis, is a disease of the aged in Western civilization. Its reported incidence is from 10% to 25% of all patients with colonic diverticulosis. Like appendicitis, it leads to intra-abdominal sepsis, with aerobic and anaerobic bacterial flora. However, the clinical manifestations of diverticulitis are more variable, the diagnosis is more difficult, and morbidity and mortality are higher than for appendicitis.

Diverticulitis is thought to be initiated by localized perforation of a diverticulum. Obstruction of the stoma of a diverticulum or high intraluminal pressure created by segmentation contraction of the colon is considered responsible for the perforation of a diverticulum. The sigmoid colon is the commonest site of diverticulitis. This finding is expected, since both segmentation contractions and diverticula are most commonly found in the sigmoid colon. Because colonic diverticula protrude into the leaves of the mesentery or appendices epiploicae, the infection is at first confined to the mesentery of the colon. Sometimes this infection is mild and resolves spontaneously. Alternatively, in about 20% of the patients, the infection may progress and lead to complications such as: (1) abscess formation; (2) free perforation; (3) obstruction; or (4) fistulization.

CLINICAL FEATURES

Typically, diverticulitis of the sigmoid colon presents with acute lower abdominal pain that localizes to the left lower quadrant or suprapubic area. The pain is usually aching in character, unremitting, and associated with fever.

Abdominal examination reveals tenderness in the left lower quadrant. Rectal examination may reveal pelvic tenderness and material testing positive for occult blood. Frank bleeding is not associated with diverticulitis. This clinical situation changes according to the severity of diverticulitis.

In patients with mild infection, pain and tenderness are mild and constitutional symptoms are few. These clinical signs and symptoms may be misdiagnosed as diverticulosis with colon spasm. White cell count elevation and fever are typical in diverticulitis and are absent in diverticulosis with spastic colon. Patients may recover rapidly from mild diverticulitis, and some may not even seek medical advice. Such unnoticed resolution of diverticulitis may explain the incidence of sigmoid colon stenosis or colovesical fistula without apparent previous diverticulitis.

Alternatively, the acute infection may be more severe, spreading beyond the confines of the sigmoid colon and its mesentery but remaining contained by adjacent organs, intestine, or omentum. Such patients experience more pain and fever and demonstrate muscle guarding and rebound tenderness in the left lower quadrant of the abdomen. These patients also suffer from nausea, vomiting, and abdominal distention resulting from the accompanying intestinal ileus. White blood cell count elevation is more pronounced, with left-shifted differential count. With hydration and appropriate antibiotic therapy, most patients make uneventful recovery. Patients who recover from uncomplicated diverticulitis are at about a 30% risk for recurrent diverticulitis. The chances for recurrence and the complication rate seem to increase with each episode of diverticulitis. Therefore, an elective sigmoid colectomy is advised after the second episode of diverticulitis.

DIAGNOSTIC IMAGING

Four views of the abdomen may reveal small-intestinal ileus, colon obstruction, free air in the peritoneal cavity, or a mass effect (displacement of intestinal gas) in the left lower quadrant. Formerly, barium or Gastrografin enema was used to diagnose diverticulitis or its complications. These studies are fraught with the danger of perforation of the colon and producing fatal barium peritonitis. Barium perforation is likely to occur in patients with acute inflammation or preexisting localized perforation, as evidenced by abdominal tenderness. The risk of perforation with contrast is increased in patients on corticosteroid therapy, even after tenderness has resolved, apparently caused by impaired healing. With the emergence of imaging studies, contrast enemas are seldom if ever used in acute diverticulitis. However, barium enema is very useful in the diagnosis of chronic fistula resulting from diverticulitis.

Computed tomography (CT) may be useful but not essential in the diagnosis of early or uncomplicated diverticulitis. At this stage, altered attenuation of the pericolic fat, indicating an inflammatory process, is seen on the CT images. The presence of very small amounts of free peritoneal air or fluid can be detected by CT, corroborating the clinical diagnosis of free perforation. The presence of a fistula or an obstructed colon may also be well delineated by CT scan. However, free perforation and obstruction of the intestine is usually quite evident clinically, and CT scan is not needed. CT scan is most useful in patients with abscess formation, where the scan can identify the number, size, and exact location of abscesses. Diverticular abscess can also be diagnosed by ultrasonography. Abscesses that are solitary and large with direct access for drainage can also be managed by percutaneous drainage with CT or ultrasonic guidance.

DIFFERENTIAL DIAGNOSIS

The initial diagnosis of acute diverticulitis is based on clinical findings. When an elderly patient presents with abdominal pain, fever, left lower quadrant abdominal tenderness, and leukocytosis, the clinical diagnosis of acute diverticulitis should be made. It should be noted that spastic sigmoid colon may be palpable as a sausage-shaped tender mass in the left lower abdominal quadrant. If a mass is not clearly detected, the tenderness alone may lead to a misdiagnosis of diverticulitis. Fever and leukocytosis are characteristic of diverticulitis and are absent when spastic colon is seen in diverticulosis without inflammation.

The inflammation localized to the left lower quadrant of the abdomen or pelvis usually seen in patients with diverticulitis may also be due to inflammation associated with ischemic colitis, Crohn's colitis, perforating carcinoma, acute appendicitis, acute salpingitis, etc. Sigmoidoscopy is valuable in the detection of mucosal abnormalities associated with ischemic colitis, ulcerative colitis, and colon carcinoma. In patients with diverticulitis, the visualized mucosa is normal. When the mucosa of the narrowed segment of the colon cannot be visualized, carcinoma of the colon may be impossible to differentiate from diverticulitis except by an operation. Acute salpingitis occurs in young women, and examinations of cervical smears may reveal intracellular gram-negative diplococci. When appendicitis is confined to the tip of a long appendix located in the left lower quadrant, it may be confused with diverticulitis. This situation is extremely unusual, but it poses the danger of delaying operation until the appendix is perforated. Acute appendicitis generally starts with epigastric pain, as opposed to the suprapubic pain seen in diverticulitis. Regardless of the etiology, worsening peritoneal infection and decision to operate for acute illness can be made by repeated clinical evaluation of the patient.

Diverticulitis may be mistaken for acute appendicitis if an inflamed sigmoid colon loop is located in the right lower quadrant. Such confusion could arise in the younger patient, especially. In this setting, early operative intervention for suspected acute appendicitis may necessitate a colostomy and staged operations for diverticulitis that otherwise might have resolved with medical management.

The most important differential diagnosis in a patient whose acute symptoms have resolved is carcinoma of the colon. Both diseases occur predominately in the older age group and present with altered bowel habits and stool positive for occult blood. Differentiation between carcinoma and diverticulitis is important, since surgical intervention should be early in carcinoma, whereas it is best delayed in diverticulitis that has resolved.

In the past, proctosigmoidoscopy was used to detect carcinoma in the visualized colon and barium enema was used to examine the rest of the colon. An intact mucosal pattern with extraluminal tracking of the barium is sufficient proof of diverticulitis. Demonstration of diverticula or signs of spastic colon, such as irregularity, thickening, and picket-fence appearance of the intestinal contour are not sufficient to diagnose diverticulitis and do not rule out carcinoma. Carcinoma generally involves a short segment of intestine, produces a shelving luminal edge and, most importantly, an abnormal mucosal pattern. Even with expert interpretation, barium enema may fail to make the distinction between carcinoma and diverticulitis.

Currently, colonoscopy is used to visualize and biopsy the mucosa in the affected segment of the colon. The diagnostic ability may be enhanced by employing the thinner gastroscope in patients with a tight stricture. On occasion, even the flexible endoscope may not be negotiable to the site of the lesion because of severe stenosis or angulation at the rectosigmoid junction. To avoid neglecting a possible carcinoma of the colon, such patients should undergo early elective surgical resection of the involved colon.

COMPLICATIONS OF DIVERTICULITIS

About 15% to 30% of the patients with diverticulitis develop complications, such as colon perforation, with generalized peritonitis, abscess formation, fistula, or colonic obstruction requiring surgical intervention.

Perforation

Perforation of the colon is reported to occur in about 14% of patients with diverticulitis resulting in diffuse peritonitis. Peritonitis may also occur with rupture of a large pericolic abscess. In either case, the patient presents with severe, acute, and diffuse abdominal pain. There is abdominal wall rigidity and the patient may be in septic shock. Rapid resuscitation and urgent laparotomy are imperative. The mortality associated with this condition may be as high as 33%.

Abscess Formation

Pericolic abscess must be suspected if pain, fever, and leukocytosis of acute diverticulitis does not improve after 48 hours of medical management. This diagnosis is more likely in patients with a tender mass in the pelvis or the left lower quadrant of the abdomen. Ultrasonography or CT scan will confirm the diagnosis of an abscess and differentiate it from a phlegmon. These imaging studies also aid in percutaneous drainage of an abscess when it is suitably located. Undetected or untreated, pericolic abscess may rupture into the peritoneal cavity, causing diffuse peritonitis, or into an adjacent viscus, resulting in a fistula. Occasionally the abscess points to the skin and when drained leads to colocutaneous fistula. There is a 6% mortality rate associated with diverticular abscess because of septic complications. Diverticular abscess should be identified and drained before serious sepsis sets in and leads to death.

Obstruction

Intestinal obstruction caused by diverticulitis may occur in both the acute and the chronic phase of the disease. In the acute phase, a loop of small intestine may be trapped in the diverticular phlegmon or abscess, leading to mechanical small-intestine obstruction. In some patients the symptoms and signs of intestinal obstruction may predominate over those of infection. Small-intestine obstruction in an elderly patient with no hernias or previous laparotomy should bring to mind an intra-abdominal abscess as a cause. Diverticulitis with a large phlegmon or abscess may also lead to acute colon obstruction. Mechanical intestinal obstruction must be differentiated from intestinal ileus, which is more common in acute diverticulitis. Four views of the abdomen may be sufficient to make this distinction. CT scan makes the diagnosis with more certainty. Barium enema, which is normally useful in the diagnosis of large-intestine obstruction, is dangerous in patients with any abdominal tenderness, since it may result in perforated colon and fatal barium peritonitis. Gastrografin enema is advocated as a safer alternative. Although perforation associated Gastrografin may be less deleterious, the advent of CT scan has obviated the need for contrast enema at all.

Recurrent attacks of diverticulitis may lead to inflammatory narrowing of a segment of the sigmoid and cause partial colon obstruction. Patients present with cramping abdominal pain, flatulence, and altered bowel habits. Patients are not acutely ill with infection, and a barium enema may be used to demonstrate the stricture under these circumstances. Colonoscopy is also a good tool for diagnosing the stricture. In addition, colonoscopic balloon dilatation can cure the stricture. Operative resection is the standard therapy for such strictures.

Fistulization

Diverticulitis may lead to fistulization between the colon and adjacent viscera such as the urinary bladder, vagina, small intestine, or the skin surface. Fistulous communication develops when a pericolic abscess ruptures into a viscus or when recurrent attacks of diverticulitis produce contiguity of surfaces and eventual necrosis of the common wall. A colovesical fistula results in the passage of feces, air, and pus in the urine. Pneumaturia (passage of air in the urine) is pathognomonic of colovesical fistula. Colovaginal and colovesical fistulas may also be caused by carcinoma, Crohn's disease, or radiation enteritis. Differential diagnosis is facilitated by cystoscopy, barium enema, CT scan, or colonoscopy. Coloenteric fistulas present with diarrhea similar to that in short bowel syndrome. Colocutaneous fistulas are not likely to heal spontaneously and therefore require surgical correction.

UNUSUAL FORMS OF DIVERTICULITIS

Unusual Location

We have so far discussed diverticulitis involving the sigmoid colon and its complications. However, colonic pseudodiverticulosis affects other parts of the colon and therefore diverticulitis may involve other parts of the colon. The clinical presentation varies, depending on the location of diverticulitis. For example, with early infection, tenderness may be located in parts of the abdomen other than the left lower quadrant. When diverticulitis is located in other parts of the colon it may be confused with peptic ulcer disease, acute cholecystitis, pancreatitis, and acute appendicitis. The correct diagnosis may therefore be delayed.

Diverticulitis in the Young

Colonic diverticulosis is uncommon in patients of less than 40 years. However, its incidence in this age group may be increasing, and age alone should not exclude this diagnosis. When it occurs in the young patient, diverticulitis is more apt to be confused with appendicitis. Diverticulitis in the young patient tends to recur with complication more often than in the elderly. Therefore, an early elective surgical intervention may be indicated in this age group.

Cecal Diverticulitis

The cecum is the site of a congenital true diverticulum possessing all three layers of the bowel wall. Inflammation of this diverticulum presents with right lower quadrant pain and tenderness and may perforate like appendicitis. The operation needed to deal with this condition is different from that for appendicitis.

SUMMARY

Diverticulitis occurs in the sigmoid colon of the elderly. Severe lower abdominal pain with fever, leukocytosis, and abdominal tenderness should suggest the diagnosis, and antibiotic therapy should be instituted in the hospital setting. About 30% of patients with diverticulitis develop life-threatening complications requiring surgical intervention. On follow-up, about a third of the patients with uncomplicated diverticulitis develop a second episode of diverticulitis with even higher complication rates. Diverticulitis mimics many conditions including colon carcinoma. Computerized tomography and colonoscopy are useful tools in the diagnosis of complications and in the differential diagnosis. Operative intervention is the mainstay of management of the complications of diverticulitis.

SUGGESTED READING

Almay TP, Howell DA. Diverticular disease of the colon. *N Engl J Med.* 1980; 302:324–331.

Pohlman T. Diverticulitis. *Gastrointest Clin North Am.* 1988; 17:357–385.

Sleisenger MH, Fordtran JS. *Gastrointestinal Disease: Pathophysiology, Diagnosis, Management.* 5th ed. Philadelphia, Pa: WB Saunders Co; 1993.

Veidenheimer MC, Roberts PL. *Colonic Diverticular Disease.* Boston, Mass: Blackwell Scientific Publications; 1991.

CHAPTER 9

■

Perforated Viscus

William D. Soper, MD

Perforation of an abdominal viscus presents the physician with an urgent diagnostic problem. The spillage of gastrointestinal contents into the abdomen can be lethal if not handled promptly. Serious morbidity and death from multiple organ failure can result from a delay in diagnosis and therapy.

Peritonitis is the common endpoint of a perforated viscus. The patient appears quite ill and lies with thighs flexed. The most common symptom is abdominal pain, which may be most intense over the area of rupture. Fever, tachycardia with a weak pulse, and abdominal distention will be present in a patient with established secondary bacterial peritonitis. Vomiting may be present with established peritonitis because of functional intestinal obstruction caused by the inflammation.

Findings on physical examination of a patient with generalized peritonitis include abdominal distention, loss of bowel sounds, generalized tenderness, guarding, and rigidity. Rectal and vaginal examination may reveal signs of pelvic peritonitis or other pathologic conditions.

A good history from the patient will often identify the problem. The character and onset of the pain are important. A perforated ulcer usually causes the sudden onset of severe pain in the epigastrium, whereas the pain of appendicitis is generally slow in onset and may actually lessen temporarily if perforation occurs. Intense pain may not occur with perforation of the bladder, although anuria and lower abdominal discomfort are usually present.

A history of previous disease may identify the source of peritonitis. Most patients with perforating duodenal or gastric ulcer relate a history of upper abdominal pain occurring several hours after eating that is relieved by food or antacids. However, 20% to 25% of patients presenting with a perforating peptic ulcer do not give a history of preceding dyspepsia. A previous history of biliary colic is often present in patients with acute cholecystitis and perforation of the gallbladder. A history of bowel irregularity and episodes of lower abdominal crampy pain may precede perforation of a sigmoid colon diverticulum. Systemic diseases such as polyarteritis nodosa, systemic lupus erythematosus, and scleroderma can cause gastroinestinal tract perforations. The patient should be asked about the ingestion of any foreign bodies. Many surgeons have removed chicken bones, fish bones, or metallic objects from sites of intestinal perforation.

The examiner should question the patient about recent or previous trauma to the abdomen or chest. Penetrating trauma is obvious, but an elderly patient may not relate a history of a fall that could have bruised or lacerated the spleen or other organ.

DIFFERENTIAL DIAGNOSIS

The differential diagnosis of abdominal peritonitis caused by a perforated viscus includes extra-abdominal, retroperitoneal, and systemic processes. Myocardial infarction and pneumonia are two important extra-abdominal processes to consider in a differential diagnosis. Myocardial infarction occasionally presents with severe epigastric pain of sudden onset, tachycardia, nausea, and vomiting. These symptoms can mislead one to the diagnosis of a perforating gastric or duodenal ulcer. An electrocardiogram and a careful history and physical examination should differentiate these conditions. Lobar pneumonia, especially in young or old patients, can present as a localized acute abdominal process. This can lead to the erroneous diagnosis of appendicitis or cholecystitis. Obviously an upright roentgenogram of the chest should be performed in all patients with abdominal pain. Free air under the diaphragm may be seen, but more importantly, a pneumonia may be revealed. The treatment of this condition is entirely different.

Acute inflammation of the pancreas and kidney in the retroperitoneal space may be difficult to differentiate from intra-abdominal peritonitis. Acute pancreatitis is discussed in Chapter 7. Acute pyelonephritis or renal colic may be confused with cholecystitis, appendicitis, perforating peptic ulcer, or another inflammatory process in the abdomen. Pyelonephritis frequently presents with abdominal pain but almost always presents with flank or midback pain. Computed tomographic (CT) scan of the abdomen is very helpful in making the diagnosis of pyelonephritis with perinephric abscess. The performance of an intravenous pyelogram should reveal a renal calculus if the pain is caused by renal colic. Urinalysis is usually abnormal in these conditions.

Several systemic illnesses may present primarily with abdominal pain and tenderness on examination. Diabetic ketoacidosis, acute intermittent porphyria, hemolytic crisis of hereditary spherocytosis or sickle cell anemia, and the gastric crisis of tabes dorsalis can all present with severe abdominal pain. Performance of good history taking and physical examination should reveal these conditions. The degree of pain related by these patients may be out of proportion to that found by physical examination. One should question the diagnosis of acute intra-abdominal peritonitis whenever the physical findings are less dramatic than those expressed by the patient.

The most helpful tests to perform in evaluating a patient with acute abdominal pain are flat plate and upright roentgenograms of the abdomen and a CT scan of the abdomen. Abdominal paracentesis and lavage can be a helpful diagnostic technique, especially in patients with blunt abdominal trauma.

There are several ways to perform a peritoneal lavage. We prefer the sterile introduction of a catheter into the peritoneal cavity through the midline beneath the umbilicus under local anesthesia. A small incision is made, exposing the peritoneum. A catheter is inserted and the contents of the abdominal cavity are aspirated. The presence of gross blood is considered a positive return and indicates the need for surgical exploration. A liter of buffered Ringer's lactate solution is introduced and then allowed to drain out under gravity. The effluent is examined for blood and debris that, if present, may aid in the diagnosis of intra-abdominal hemorrhage or intestinal perforation. Peritoneal lavage is of no real value in a patient with diffuse peritonitis. This patient needs fluid resuscitation and laparotomy.

One should examine the patient after giving morphine for pain or after induction of anesthesia before laparotomy. The presence of an abdominal mass or fullness may alter the diagnostic and operative approach.

PERFORATING GASTRIC OR DUODENAL ULCER

Perforation of a peptic ulcer causes the acute onset of severe epigastric pain. The pain is intense, unrelenting, and rapidly spreads throughout the abdomen. Pain felt at the top of the shoulder indicates that the spillage of the gastric contents has spread to the diaphragm. Nausea and vomiting may occur but are not constant findings.

Physical examination reveals an acutely ill patient in marked distress who is lying immobile, often with the thighs flexed. Respirations are shallow and grunting. The abdomen is rigid, with generalized tenderness that is maximal in the epigastrium. Bowel sounds are usually absent. Mild tachycardia is usually present and the pulse may be weak.

The findings at this stage of the illness are mainly the result of reflex mechanisms caused by the chemical irritation of the anterior peritoneum. The area of peritonitis rapidly enlarges as the gastric and duodenal fluid flows through the perforation. Rectal and pelvic examinations at this time will often show a fullness or tenderness in the pouch of Douglas. This indicates the presence of caustic gastric fluid in the pelvis. However, sometimes the fluid localizes to the right lower quadrant because of the presence of the falciform ligament and right colon. The presence of free air in the peritoneal cavity is indicated by tympany to percussion and loss of the normal liver dullness laterally and anteriorly. Shifting dullness, if present, suggests free intraperi-toneal fluid.

If peritoneal soiling continues for 8 to 12 hours, a secondary bacterial peritonitis may develop. The patient will now have a fever and abdominal distention. He or she may actually lose the muscular rigidity because of the toxic effect of sepsis on the neuromuscular system. The release of histamine and other vasoactive substances in the peritoneal cavity causes a massive ex-udation of plasma into the abdomen. This produces distention and causes hy-povolemia, hypotension, and tachycardia. Gram-positive and gram-negative bacteria may translocate through the intestinal wall, causing a bacterial peritonitis. Antibiotic coverage should be broad and directed at these organ-isms.

Diagnosis is not difficult. The patient often gives a history of previous ul-cer symptoms that have exacerbated in the 2 to 3 days before perforation. A chest radiograph and electrocardiogram rule out clinically significant car-diopulmonary disease. Flat plate and upright radiographs of the abdomen and chest show free air in the peritoneal cavity in more than 50% of patients. Complete blood count shows a moderate leukocytosis of 14 000 to 16 000 white blood cells within a few hours of perforation and a left shift of the white blood cell differential. The hematocrit value increases as the plasma volume decreases with intra-abdominal exudation of fluid. The serum amylase may be mildly elevated but is usually less than 200 Somogyi units and rarely ex-ceeds 600 units.

Occasionally the diagnosis may be in doubt, even after a complete his-tory and physical examination and review of the laboratory data. If free air was not demonstrated on upright examination of the abdomen, a CT scan of the abdomen with oral contrast can help establish the diagnosis of perfora-tion of the stomach or duodenum. On occasion an esophagogastroduo-denogram using a water-soluble dye such as Gastrografin may demonstrate the perforation (Fig. 33).

Occasionally gastric and duodenal ulcers do not perforate into the free peritoneal cavity but instead rupture posteriorly into the lesser sac or the retroperitoneum. A gastric ulcer that perforates into the lesser sac will cause a sudden onset of pain. The pain is often less intense and is referred to the back. However, if fluid escapes through the foramen of Winslow into the main peri-toneal cavity, the classic findings of a perforating ulcer will occur. Posterior per-foration of a duodenal ulcer can present with acute hemorrhage into the stom-ach and duodenum from erosion of pancreatic vessels. Pain is again mainly felt in the back, and the symptoms and signs of free perforation are absent.

Another variation in clinical presentation results from the early cessation of leakage of gastric contents. A small perforation may seal spontaneously by fibrinous fusion to the quadrate lobe of the liver, gallbladder, and falciform ligament. The patient experiences upper abdominal pain of short duration. Physical findings are not severe and may disappear rapidly. However, free air

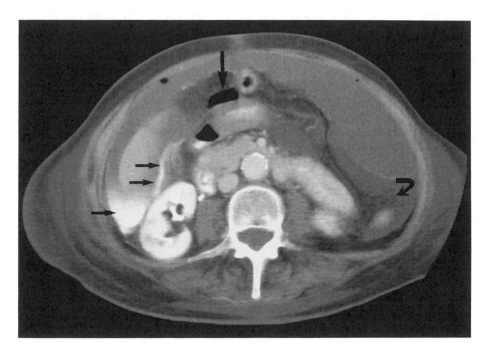

Figure 33. Contrast-enhanced computed tomogram of the abdomen of a patient complaining of abdominal pain. Plain abdominal radiographs were nonspecific. Note the free air beneath the liver (large arrow), spillage of oral contrast medium from the duodenum into the right paracolic space (small arrows), and free peritoneal fluid (curved arrow). At laparotomy a perforated duodenal ulcer was identified.

may still be present in the peritoneal cavity, establishing the diagnosis of a contained (forme fruste) perforation.

The differential diagnosis has already been discussed. One must especially consider acute cholecystitis, acute pancreatitis, myocardial infarction, and if the symptoms occur predominantly in the right lower quadrant, acute appendicitis. The main concern, however, is to determine if a surgical or non-surgical condition exists. The cause of the abdominal pain will remain obscure until surgical exploration reveals the problem.

PERFORATION OF THE SMALL INTESTINE

Intestinal wounds are created by a variety of mechanisms. External trauma of either a blunt or penetrating variety is the most common cause. Blunt trauma (crushing injuries, deceleration injuries, a blow from a fist or club, or a fall

146 / CHAPTER 9

from a height) may create a severe contusion, causing perforation of the intestinal wall at one or more points. Penetrating wounds are most commonly gunshot wounds or knife wounds. Trauma also can be of an internal variety. Ingested foreign bodies such as shells, toothpicks, bone fragments, pins, or other obscure foreign objects can perforate the intestine from the inside out. Prolonged distention from an intestinal obstruction with areas of localized gangrene can progress to perforation. Certain infectious diseases may cause perforation of the small intestine. Most of these diseases, such as tuberculosis and cytomegalovirus infections occur in immunocompromised patients.

PERFORATION OF THE COLON

Perforation of the colon is often fatal, especially if it occurs in elderly patients. Therefore, diagnosis and treatment must proceed rapidly. The second most common cause of free air in the peritoneal cavity is perforation of the colon. Gastroduodenal perforation is the most common cause. Diverticulitis is the most common cause of perforation of the colon and is present in 40% to 50% of patients with a perforated colon. The colon is a rich source of bacteria and thus the peritonitis associated with perforation of a colonic diverticulum is bacterial from the onset. *Escherichia coli* and *Bacteroides* species are the bacteria most commonly cultured from the abdomen after colonic perforations. Broad-spectrum antibiotics must be administered early in the clinical course to help control the infection.

Acute diverticulitis with perforation occurs most frequently in the sigmoid and descending colon. The incidence of diverticulitis and perforation increases with age and is rarely found in patients younger than 40 years. Most patients are in their fifth to seventh decade of life and often give a history of previous left lower quadrant abdominal pain of varying severity. The pain is usually described as cramping in nature. Chronic constipation is another frequent complaint in these patients. The acute episode of diverticulitis often begins as a sudden onset of or increase in left lower quadrant pain. Nausea and vomiting are not early findings but may occur later with diffuse peritonitis. Free perforation probably occurs in less than 5% of diverticular attacks, although contained perforation may occur in up to 50% of instances of diverticulitis.

Physical examination reveals a patient in acute distress, often holding his or her lower abdomen. Most patients are moderately febrile, with a fever of 102° to 103°F. Bowel sounds disappear quickly. Maximal tenderness is located over the site of perforation. Generalized tenderness with guarding and rebound tenderness will be present if free contamination of the peritoneal cavity has occurred. Loss of the normal liver dullness to percussion over the anterolateral aspect of the liver suggests the presence of free air. Rectovaginal examination may reveal a mass in the pelvis, with maximal tenderness on the left side. A mass also may be palpable transabdominally, but often the abdominal muscles are too tense to allow accurate definition of an abscess. The treatment of perforating diverticulitis with generalized peritonitis is surgical and should not be delayed. Fluid resuscitation can be started while the patient is evaluated for any coexisting diseases, such as heart failure.

Occasionally the colon may perforate into an adjoining viscus such as the vagina or urinary bladder. The patient may note the passage of gas or feculent material from the vagina or with urination. Proper management of these complicated fistulas requires diagnostic evaluations that can be done leisurely, as colovaginal and colovesical fistulas are not surgical emergencies.

Other disease processes may cause perforations of the colon. Carcinoma, ischemic colitis, ulcerative colitis, amebic colitis, cecal or sigmoid volvulus, foreign body penetration, stercoral ulceration, and spontaneous rupture are a few of the processes to consider in a differential diagnosis of colonic perforations.

The immunocompromised patient presents a difficult diagnostic problem and represents an ever-growing segment of the patient population. These patients may be receiving chemotherapeutic agents to treat cancers, have undergone organ or tissue transplantation, or may have human immunodeficiency virus (HIV) infections. It is common for these patients who are severely immunocompromised to develop acute abdominal pain. A CT scan of the abdomen may be very helpful in finding the cause of the pain (see Chapter 15).

PERFORATION OF THE ESOPHAGUS

Spontaneous rupture of the esophagus, Boerhaave's syndrome, is the most serious perforation of the gastrointestinal tract. Morbidity and mortality increase dramatically if diagnosis and treatment occur longer than 12 hours from the time of perforation. The classic clinical presentation is one of forceful vomiting followed by mild hematemesis and substernal chest pain. The pain is the most striking feature and is pleuritic in the left chest and radiates to the epigastrium, substernal region, or back. Dysphagia is present. Dyspnea occurs quickly and the patient has rapid and shallow respirations because of the excruciating pain. Occasionally the presence of epigastric pain and tenderness may suggest the diagnosis of perforating gastric or duodenal ulcer. However, as the disease progresses, the abdominal signs of rigidity and tenderness often lessen, while the thoracic signs increase. Spontaneous pneumothorax and palpable crepitus in the suprasternal notch or neck may develop.

The diagnosis is made on a chest roentgenogram that will show a left pneumothorax and pleural effusion. If any doubt remains, a Gastrografin esophagogram will reveal contrast in the left chest in about 70% of patients. Endoscopy is of no value and may be harmful.

RUPTURE OF THE GALLBLADDER AND BILE DUCTS

The gallbladder and bile ducts may rupture after blunt trauma to the abdomen or during an attack of acute cholecystitis. Perforation occurs in 3% to 10% of instances of acute cholecystitis and may be one of three types:

Type 1. Free perforation with bile peritonitis.
Type 2. Subacute perforation with local abscess.
Type 3. Chronic perforation with cholecystenteric fistula.

Patients with biliary tract perforations are often older and have systemic diseases, such as atherosclerotic vascular disease, malignant tumors, or systemic lupus erythematosus. The clinical symptoms are the same as for acute cholecystitis, except the illness is slower to respond to treatment. Pain, fever, and anorexia persist for several days after the initial symptoms occur. However, if a Type 1 perforation is present, diffuse peritonitis will be present early and the diagnosis will become obvious.

Rupture of the biliary ducts is reported but is not common. The entire biliary tract is usually diseased, and chronic or acute cholecystitis is also present. The diagnosis of a perforation of the bile ducts is rarely made preoperatively. The pathologic condition is found during exploration for symptoms consistent with cholecystitis or perforation of the gallbladder. Occasionally congenital choledochal cysts of the common bile duct may rupture during pregnancy or labor, producing acute abdominal pain. A more common cause of rupture of the bile ducts today is either penetrating or blunt trauma to the upper abdomen involving the liver or head of the pancreas.

LIVER ABSCESS

Primary liver abscesses are rare in the United States. They are often caused by an intra-abdominal infection such as perforated appendix or diverticulitis or, most commonly, in association with cholangitis. Amebic liver abscess is common in some parts of the world and in the United States occurs more frequently in southern than northern states. Amebic liver abscess also can occur in any person who has recently traveled to areas where amebiasis is endemic or who is a resident or a chronic care facility. The patient will usually have a spiking fever of 100° to 105°F, malaise, anorexia, weakness, weight loss, and abdominal distention. Pain is frequently present and is dull and constant over the liver. Deep inspiration will cause pleuritic pain if diaphragmatic involvement is present. Enlargement and tenderness of the liver are constant physical findings. Liver abscess is one of the few conditions that can produce upward enlargement of the liver. Mild jaundice is common. Free perforation will produce signs of peritonitis. However, abdominal rigidity is not a constant finding in perforated amebic liver abscess. Amebic abscess and peritonitis should be suspected if the patient is male and has had a recent history of diarrhea and any possible exposure to *Entamoeba histolytica*. Flat plate roentgenograms of the abdomen may show a speckled gas pattern in the liver, gallbladder, or bile ducts. Chest roentgenograms are abnormal 50% of the time, showing elevation of the right hemidiaphragm, pleural effusion, and right-sided atelectasis. Abdominal CT scan identifies a liver abscess.

PERFORATION OF THE APPENDIX

The classic symptoms of anorexia followed by midabdominal pain that localizes to the right lower quadrant leads to the diagnosis of acute appendicitis. However, the atypical case may present with perforation and all the signs of localized or generalized peritonitis. In about 5% of patients with perforated appendicitis, a small amount of air may appear under the diaphragm. However, if a large amount of free air is present, the diagnosis of perforated appendix should be doubted and a perforation of the colon suspected.

PERFORATION OF THE URINARY BLADDER

Perforation of the bladder is most often associated with trauma to the pelvis. A bone fragment can penetrate the bladder during a crush injury of the pelvis. Gunshot wounds and stab wounds may injure the bladder. Blunt trauma in the form of a blow just above the pubic bone may rupture a distended bladder but generally not an empty bladder. An intravenous pyelogram and cystogram should be performed in all patients with abdominal or pelvic trauma before surgical exploration.

Tumors, tuberculosis, and prostatic obstruction may also predispose the bladder to rupture. Symptoms of pelvic peritonitis with pain, guarding, rigidity, and ileus may occur soon after the injury. However, the injury may not produce symptoms for some time if sterile urine is slowly leaking into the peritoneal cavity. Oliguria, abdominal ascites, and lower abdominal discomfort may suggest the diagnosis. A cystogram usually, but not always, shows the perforation. Physical findings and clinical suspicion may be the only clue to the diagnosis.

RUPTURED OVARY

Mittelschmerz is the pain associated with ovulation and is a common cause of abdominal pain in women. The pain may be mild and transient or may be severe enough to be confused with acute appendicitis if present on the right side of the abdomen. Ovulation releases a small amount of blood into the abdominal cavity and this blood irritates the peritoneum. The pain occurs in the middle of the menstrual cycle. It presents lower in the pelvis than McBurney's point and is not accompanied by anorexia or nausea. The ovary, if palpable, will usually be tender. However, the clinical picture just described can vary in severity and time of occurrence in the menstrual cycle, leading to the diagnosis of pelvic peritonitis requiring laparoscopy or laparotomy. It is far better to operate when faced with such a confusing clinical presentation and remove a normal appendix than to wait, only to be forced to drain an appendiceal abscess later.

Rupture of a corpus luteum cyst does not usually produce significant abdominal pain. However, if the cyst is large and rupture is accompanied by bleeding, the patient may present with acute pelvic peritonitis and shock. Rupture of the cyst can follow physical exercise or sexual intercourse. Nausea and vomiting occur soon after the onset of pain. The pain continues to be constant and dull, initially confined to one side of the lower abdomen. Generalized lower abdominal pain occurs if enough intraperitoneal contamination occurs with cyst fluid and blood. The pain is almost always confined to the lower abdomen. Guarding and rigidity of the lower abdominal muscles can occur. Pelvic examination will usually localize the side of greatest tenderness and may reveal a fullness. Pelvic ultrasonographic examination will show free fluid in the pelvis. Culdocentesis (needle aspiration of the cul-de-sac) will reveal blood and cyst fluid. If bleeding is minimal and stops early, the pain will gradually fade away, leaving the patient with some lower abdominal soreness and discomfort for several days. However, if the bleeding continues, the pain progresses, tachycardia and hypotension occur, and exploration is required.

RUPTURED FALLOPIAN TUBES

Tubo-ovarian abscess and ectopic pregnancy are conditions of the fallopian tubes that can rupture, causing acute abdominal symptoms. Tubo-ovarian abscess results from infection in the fallopian tubes that spreads to involve the pelvic peritoneum, ovary, and tube in an abscess process. The patient often has high, spiking fevers and localized pelvic peritonitis with a mass palpable on pelvic examination. Rupture of the abscess can cause the development of shock, tachycardia, and spreading peritonitis in the abdomen. Immediate operative treatment is indicated.

Rupture of a tubal pregnancy may present with acute abdominal pain, shock, tachycardia, nausea, vomiting, and abdominal distention. Emergency surgical exploration is necessary to control the hemorrhage and save the patient's life. Few tests will be helpful in establishing this diagnosis. A history of a missed menstrual period in a sexually active woman with the clinical signs and symptoms of shock and pelvic peritonitis is all that is needed to suspect the diagnosis of ruptured ectopic pregnancy. Pelvic ultrasonography may show the tubal pregnancy with free fluid around the tube, and a pregnancy test will be positive.

SUGGESTED READING

Asensio JA, Weigelt JA, eds. Contemporary problems in trauma surgery. *Surg Clin North Am.* 1991; 71:209–433.

Delany HM, Jason RS. *Abdominal Trauma: Surgical and Radiologic Diagnosis.* Berlin, Germany: Springer-Verlag; 1981.

Federle MP, ed. Radiology of the immunocompromised patient. *Radiol Clin North Am.* 1993; 30:507–659.

Jeffrey RB, Jr. *CT and Sonography of the Acute Abdomen.* New York, NY: Raven Press; 1989.

Sawyers JL, Williams LF, eds. The acute abdomen. *Surg Clin North Am.* 1988; 68:233–471.

Thal ER, ed. Abdominal trauma. *Surg Clin North Am.* 1990; 70:495–733 .

Williamson RCN, Cooper MJ. *Emergency Abdominal Surgery.* Edinburgh, Scotland: Churchill Livingstone; 1990.

CHAPTER 10

■

Intestinal Obstruction

Charles Aprahamian, MD

When a patient presents with pain, nausea, vomiting, abdominal distention with tympania, hyperactive bowel sounds, and obstipation several questions must be asked.

DOES THE PATIENT HAVE AN INTESTINAL OBSTRUCTION?

Colicky pain results from peristalsis in any muscular tubular structure with partial or complete obstruction. The patient may not appreciate the meaning of *colicky* but recognizes the phrase "cramps" or the significance of the examiner demonstrating the gripping pain by slowly clenching the fist. Parous women understand uterine contractions and can equate colicky pain with them.

With complete obstruction of the gastrointestinal (GI) tract, the patient develops obstipation, vomiting, and abdominal distention. The bowel contents distal to the obstruction may be evacuated, suggesting that bowel function is normal. However, once the intestine is completely evacuated, obstipation is noted. Intestine contents proximal to the obstruction frequently "back up" and produce a sense of fullness, nausea, and vomiting. The vomitus consists of small-intestinal contents, which may be golden in color and malodorous from bacterial overgrowth. When the suction bottle is examined, the nasogastric aspirate contains sediment. While consistently present, the abdominal distention associated with intestinal obstruction may vary in amount because emesis and nasogastric aspiration may reduce the liquid and gases that cause the distention. Frequently, the more proximal the obstruction the less the distention. Proximal jejunal obstruction causes upper-abdominal distention, whereas distal ileal obstruction results in distention of the entire abdomen. A partial obstruction may permit less than normal intestinal function and thus modify the presenting symptoms, physical signs, and adjuvant testing.

The physical examination should be directed toward making the diagnosis of intestinal obstruction and if possible to identify its cause. Abdominal distention arouses suspicion. The presence of intestinal gas will produce tympany on percussion. On ausculation, the presence of peristaltic rushes coincidental with pain secures the diagnosis. Prolonged intestinal obstruction may present with a silent abdomen, suggesting an ileus, especially if ausculation yields "tinkling" bowel sounds. Since adhesions are the most common cause of intestinal obstruction, a close examination of the abdomen for a scar leads one to this possible cause. The presence of masses in hernia sites suggests another etiology. Epigastric, umbilical, incisional, and inguinal areas should be scanned visually and palpated for a mass. Femoral hernias may result in groin masses below the inguinal ligament. Since the femoral vein is adjacent to the femoral canal, the presenting symptom may be that of lower-extremity venous occlusive disease. Another important feature of hernias is that only a portion of the intestine may become incarcerated (Richter's hernia) resulting in only a partial obstruction without evidence of a hernial mass. A similar elusive hernia is one resulting from an unsuspected previous diaphragmatic injury and defect.

Intestinal obstruction secondary to tumorous masses can also be suspected on physical examination. The palpable mass may be the primary lesion or represent metastasis. Frequently, rectal carcinomas are palpated within reach of the examining finger. Vaginal examination may demonstrate varying stages of cervical carcinoma. Metastatic intra-abdominal tumors may be palpated in the posterior fornix of the vagina, as well as in the rectal pouch. Abdominal masses could be an intestinal carcinoma. The ileocecal intussusception, from whatever cause, may be palpated as a right-sided linear tumor mass. Currant jelly stools represent bloody mucus and suggest an obstruction (intussusception). Palpable lesions of the liver or umbilicus may represent tumor metastasis. Even a palpable left scalene node could represent tumor spread from the pancreas or stomach.

Clinical evidence of intestinal obstruction in the presence of septic clinical signs and symptoms could indicate inflammation (diverticulitis) or an ischemic complication resulting from obstruction, ie, gangrene.

Radiologic testing supplements the clinical examination. The standard abdominal series includes a chest roentgenogram, flat plate, and upright of the abdomen. An abnormal chest roentgenogram may explain some of the patient's symptoms. Four of the five lung lobes are adjacent to the diaphragm, and pneumonia may produce referred abdominal pain and irritation through the intercostal nerves (8 through 12) which also innervate the abdomen. The chest roentgenogram may also demonstrate free air and perhaps a diaphragmatic defect with abdominal viscera in the left chest. The combined flat plate and upright may demonstrate air–fluid levels, gaseous outline of dilated or distended bowel, or the absence of gas in all or distal portions of the colon. Sigmoid or cecal volvulus is recognized from a characteristic colonic air pattern. The combination of a clinical and radiologic picture of obstruction with air in the biliary tree suggest a gallstone ileus. However, the same situation in a patient previously operated on may represent a simple intestinal obstruction occurring in a patient with a surgically created cholodochoduodenostomy. Radiologic contrast studies may help differentiate. Many believe proctoscopic examination to be an integral part of the physical examination. In any event, it should precede the placement of barium per rectum. The proctoscopic examination can identify an obstructing tumor mass and make the emergency barium study unnecessary. In the suspected sigmoid volvulus, proctoscopic examination may serve not only to confirm the torsion but to decompress the colon and convert an acute problem of intestinal obstruction to one of a chronic redundant colon. The patient with a radiographic picture of large- and small-intestinal gas compatible with an obstruction is benefited by a barium enema. This may clearly establish a diagnosis of large-intestinal obstruction over small-intestinal obstruction and help develop the plan of action. The barium enema can be therapeutic by reducing an ileocecal intussusception.

Patients suspected of a small-intestinal obstruction may have their diagnosis confirmed with oral contrast consisting of Gastrografin and barium. Contrast present in the colon after 2 hours of ingesting contrast indicates an open or partially open small intestine, while failure to pass it into the colon suggests an obstruction to flow.

IS THE INTESTINAL OBSTRUCTION MECHANICAL OR FUNCTIONAL?

Mechanical obstruction is caused by adhesions, hernias, tumors, inflammatory strictures, anastomotic stenosis, etc. These occlusions may be intraluminal or extraluminal, representing congenital or acquired lesions. The absence of an obvious mechanical cause in an obstructive situation represents a functional obstruction and has been called ileus. Ileus has been reported associated with medications or following both intra-abdominal and extra-abdominal operative procedures. Because ileus represents a functional obstruction, it is a diagnosis of exclusion. The clinical picture of abdominal distention, obstipation, nausea, and vomiting with radiologic evidence of air in the entire GI tract occurring in the postoperative patient is most likely ileus and should be treated supportively. If the condition persists, it demands an evaluation similar to that of the patient with the signs and symptoms of mechanical intestinal obstruction. Periodically the patient with ileus will develop progressive colonic dilatation, which has been called pseudo-obstruction. Clinically significant dilatation is manifested by right colon enlargement. Early recognition and treatment with colon decompression may avert the ischemic changes that may result in cecal perforation. Dilatation of the cecum and transverse colon of 10 and 8 cm respectively should be an indicator for action.

IS AN EMERGENCY OPERATION INDICATED?

There is no indication for an emergency operation for intestinal obstruction unless there is evidence of ischemia and of dead intestine. Even then the patient must be resuscitated first. The problem with intestinal obstruction is the hypovolemia and the metabolic changes associated with decreased oral intake, obligate urinary losses, and subsequent losses from vomiting and fluid shifts. Resuscitative activities aimed at correcting acid–base imbalances and normalization of renal function may preclude early radiologic assessment or be coincidental with it. Therefore, once the diagnosis has been confirmed, the patient's condition may be optimum for an operation, if indicated. An urgent operation is indicated when the obstruction has been complicated by ischemia. Dying and dead intestine must be removed. The presence of peritoneal signs—tenderness and guarding—and systemic evidence of sepsis (fever, tachycardia, and abnormal white cell count consisting of a left shift with or without leukocytosis) indicate the need for an early operation. In the absence of these findings, the patient could be provided with intravenous alimentation and undergo more deliberate evaluation in preparation for an abdominal operation.

The role of GI decompression deserves comment. Most of the air in the stomach is either swallowed or induced with efforts at bag-face-mask ventilation. The short tube for nasogastric intubation is easily placed and is useful in decompressing the stomach of air and liquids. It is also quite useful for the patient experiencing nausea and vomiting. A patent tube that is not removing fluid may be a discomfort to the patient, as well as being hazardous by causing erosions at the gastroesophageal junction and fostering esophageal reflux. The short tube is characterized by either a single or double lumen. The single-lumen tube should be placed on intermittent suction, whereas the double-lumen or sump tube demands continuous suction if it is to function as a sump.

A long tube for nasointestinal intubation is designed to decompress intestinal liquids and gas when present. Advocates suggest that the three indications for long-tube intubation are: (1) intestinal obstruction in a terminally ill patient when decompression may provide comfort and relief from symptoms; (2) ileus or when decompression of the small intestine is desirable; and (3) a previous presentation with "bowel obstruction" and a benefit from long-tube use.

Whereas the short tube is easy to place, the long tube is not. Patients with some peristaltic activity may benefit from a Miller-Abbott tube. This is a double-lumen tube with one of the lumens used to suction intestinal contents and the second to instill air or mercury into a balloon located at the catheter tip. This balloon serves as a bolus for the peristaltic wave. In the absence of peristalsis, eg, ileus, mercury may serve as the weight necessary to "drag" the tube through the intestines. The Cantor tube is a single-lumen long tube designed specifically for this condition. Mercury, 1.5 to 2 mL, is placed directly into the balloon attached to the catheter tip and the mercury-containing balloon catheter is inserted through the nares into the stomach. The advancement of long tubes from the stomach into the jejunum may be fostered by positional changes or fluoroscopic manipulation. The difficulty of getting the long tube to pass into the intestine may be responsible for its infrequent use.

SUGGESTED READING

Brolin RE, Krasna MJ, Mast BA. Use of tubes and radiographs in the management of small bowel obstruction. 1987; *Ann Surg.* 206:126.

James RS. Intestinal obstruction. In: Sabiston DC, ed. *Textbook of Surgery.* WB Saunders Co; Philadelphia, Pa: 1991.

Menzies D. Peritoneal adhesions: incidence, causes. *Surg Annu.* 1992; 24:27.

Nelson IW, Ellis H. The sprectum of intestinal obstruction today. *Br J Clin Pract.* 1984; 28:249.

Seror D, Feigin E, Szold A, et al. How conservatively can postoperative small bowel obstruction be treated? *Am J Surg.* 1993; 165:121.

Shackelford RT. Surgical disorders of the jejuno-ileum. In: Shackelford, RT, ed. *Diagnosis of Surgical Disease.* WB Saunders Co; Philadelphia, Pa: 1968.

CHAPTER 11

■

Mesenteric Ischemia

Jonathan B. Towne, MD

Mesenteric ischemia remains a diagnostic and therapeutic challenge for the clinicians. Despite advances in diagnostic modalities, including computed tomographic (CT) scanning, digital subtraction angiography, and more recently, magnetic resonance (MR) angiography, mesenteric ischemia has continued to be difficult to diagnose. There are several reasons for this. Mesenteric ischemia is an etiology of the acute abdomen in only 1% to 2% of patients. Because of the rarity of this diagnosis, no one physician or surgical group sees a large enough number of these patients to finely tune diagnostic and treatment algorithms.

The onset of this disease is often insidious, characterized by vague and poorly localized abdominal complaints. In addition, these patients often have advanced atherosclerotic cardiovascular disease, which has resulted in acute myocardial infarction, congestive heart failure, and end-stage atherosclerotic occlusive disease. Finally, the mesenteric circulation is impossible to assess by physical examination. The origins of the mesenteric artery arise in the midaortic segment, which is far removed from the palpating hand. The venous circulation exits via the liver, which likewise makes it impossible to see any of the usual stigmata of venous occlusive disease that are so easily seen in the upper or lower extremities or the head and neck region.

The treatment of mesenteric ischemia is also fraught with failure. Contemporary series have mortality rates that range from 60% to 80%.

ANATOMIC CONSIDERATIONS

All the mesenteric vessels arise from the abdominal aorta. Shortly after the abdominal aorta exits from the aortic hiatus of the diaphragm, it gives rise to the celiac artery. The celiac artery, in turn, has three branches, the first of which is the left gastric. The second branch is the hepatic artery, and the largest branch of the three is the splenic artery. Early arborization of the celiac axis makes it difficult for emboli to lodge anywhere beyond the initial 2 to 3 cm of this vessel. The second major mesenteric branch is the superior mesenteric artery, which usually arises approximately 1 to 2 cm caudal to the celiac artery at the level of the first lumbar vertebra. Its origin is hidden by the neck of the pancreas. As the artery emerges underneath the pancreas, it gives rise to the inferior pancreatic duodenal artery, which is the main source of collateral anastomosis with the celiac artery. Finally, the third and least significant mesenteric branch is the inferior mesenteric artery, which primarily supplies the left and sigmoid colon and provides collateral connections with the hypogastric vessels through the middle and inferior rectal arteries.

The main collaterals between the inferior mesenteric (IMA) and superior mesenteric arteries (SMA) are two. The marginal artery of Drummond runs parallel to the mesenteric border of the left colon and at the splenic flexure connects the left branch of the middle colic artery, a branch of the SMA, with the ascending branch of the left colic artery, a branch of the IMA. The meandering mesenteric artery is a large collateral that runs more centrally in the mesentery and connects the left branch of the middle colic (SMA) with the IMA.

Almost all the venous drainage of the intestine is to the portal system, which is formed at the level of the second lumbar vertebra by the junction of the superior mesenteric and splenic veins. The collateral anastomoses between the arterial branches of these three mesenteric vessels are well developed, so it is unusual for ischemic intestinal symptoms to develop with atherosclerotic occlusive disease unless two of the three mesenteric vessels are obstructed. This does not apply to the development of symptoms related to emboli because the acute nature of the occlusive emboli does not allow collateral circulation to develop. A single acutely occluded vessel can result in significant intestinal ischemia.

THE PATHOPHYSIOLOGY OF MESENTERIC ISCHEMIA

The amount of blood that goes to the intestine is distributed disproportionately. The small intestine receives one and a half to two times more blood flow per unit weight than the colon or the stomach. The mucosa and submucosa receive 70% of the flow. Within the mucosa, approximately half of the mucosal flow goes to the superficial villous region, which is the primary absorptive site. When blood flow to the intestine is reduced acutely, there is a differential effect on flow to different layers. Acute reductions in perfusion pressure, as seen with acute mesenteric embolus, are compensated by local regulatory mechanisms that lessen the effect of the hypotension, primarily by decreasing peripheral resistance. This autoregulatory mechanism is protective, allowing minor changes in nutritive blood flow with moderate reductions in blood pressure. With progression of ischemia, the intramural blood flow distributes itself primarily to the mucosa and, most importantly, to the superficial portion of the mucosa. In an etiologic sense, this is probably reasonable, in that it is the mucosa that provides the barrier between the bacteria-laden contents of the intestine and the portal venous circulation.

At the cellular level, tissue oxygen extraction increases with reduced blood flow. Obviously, when blood flow drops below a critical level, ischemic damage occurs. During the ischemic period, cellular adenosine triphosphate (ATP) is depleted, with the formation of adenosine monophosphate (AMP), which is further metabolized to adenosine, inosine, and hypoxanthine. Similarly, xanthine dehydrogenase is converted to xanthine oxidase in ischemic tissue. With reperfusion reoxygenation, superoxide radicals are produced. Xanthine oxidase and hypoxanthine combine with oxygen to form oxygen free radicals, which can cause further tissue damage during reperfusion. The intestinal mucosa is characterized by having the highest concentration of xanthine dehydrogenase in the mucosa villi and is therefore more prone to injury during reperfusion.

In the research laboratory, the toxic effect of superoxide radicals can be experimentally modulated using oxygen scavenger molecules, such as superoxide dismutase, dimethyl sulfide, and dextran, which combine with and inactivate these oxygen radicals. The mucosa is exquisitely sensitive to ischemia, and electron-microscopic changes can be seen after periods of ischemia as short as 10 minutes. More classic light microscopic histologic changes can be seen in mucosa after 1 hour of ischemia. In general, a period of 30 minutes of ischemia is required for extensive abnormalities to occur.

As the ischemic insult progresses, hemorrhage into the mesenteric vascular bed occurs, resulting in the classical features in mesenteric infarction. The intestinal wall is swollen and infiltrated with blood, the mucosa becomes necrotic, and bacterial peritonitis is present. Histologically, there is hemorrhagic necrosis with extensive submucosal edema. With the loss of mucosal integrity, bacteria can invade the layers of the intestinal wall and be carried by portal venous flow into the liver and, subsequently, into the general circulation.

CLINICAL PRESENTATION

There are four distinct types of mesenteric ischemia: arterial embolus (most commonly to the SMA), atherosclerotic occlusive disease, nonocclusive intestinal ischemia, and venous infarction. The most notable aspect of mesenteric ischemia is the absence of clinical physical findings and the disparity between the patient's symptoms and clinical findings. Classically, acute mesenteric ischemia presents as a patient writhing in bed from exquisite abdominal pain with a soft abdomen and the absence of any peritoneal findings. The uninitiated physician can mistakenly feel that the patient is malingering.

The clinical history of the patient is important. If a patient has chronic atrial fibrillation, has recently had a myocardial infarction, or has a history of a long-standing ventricular aneurysm, the possibility of embolus should be entertained. Likewise, the clinical history should be carefully taken to note if the patient has had previous, milder soft signs of mesenteric ischemia. These consist of nonspecific abdominal pain, particularly in reference to eating heavy meals. Classically, pain begins approximately 2 hours after eating. Often the episode of mesenteric ischemia is accompanied by vomiting or diarrhea, as the intestine in its earliest phases of ischemia can be quite irritable. This is often followed by a quiet abdomen with the absence of bowel sounds. The lack of peritoneal findings is due in part to the fact that in the early stages of mesenteric ischemia, movement of bacteria into the wall of the intestine causes visceral pain, which presents as nonspecific periumbilical pain. The finding of parietal peritoneal irritation is a late sign of mesenteric ischemia and is often only detected in a dying patient.

LABORATORY TESTS

An increased white count, in the range of 15 000/mm^3, is often the earliest finding. If there has been extensive movement of interstitial fluid into the wall of the intestine, hemoconcentration can be an early finding. As the intestinal wall becomes more hemorrhagic, the hematocrit falls and relative anemia can be seen. Metabolic acidosis is a common early finding. As the ischemic episode progresses and with development of increased permeability of the intestine to its contents, amylase is absorbed from the lumen and results in an elevated serum amylase level. Late in the course of mesenteric infarction, L-lactate dehydrogenase (LDH), serum glutamic-oxaloacetic transaminase (SGOT), serum glutamate pyruvate transaminase (SGPT), and creatine phosphokinase (CPK) are markedly elevated.

Plain radiographs of the abdomen should be obtained, primarily to rule out other causes of acute abdominal pain; plain radiographs are negative early in this disease. CT scanning early in the disease is likewise usually not diagnostic. However, its unique role is in diagnosing mesenteric venous occlusion, which is often easily seen on CT scans obtained with contrast. Angiography is the definitive diagnostic test for acute mesenteric ischemia. It is important that both anterior-posterior and lateral views are obtained. The angiographic findings are generally related to the cause of the thrombosis. Mesenteric artery thrombosis primarily involves the origin of the mesenteric artery and extends distally for varying distances. On the other hand, SMA emboli generally lodge at a branch point, often sparing the proximal branches of the SMA. Diffuse tapering of branches of the SMA suggests nonocclusive mesenteric ischemia.

Superior Mesenteric Emboli

Mesenteric artery emboli present with acute onset of abdominal pain, usually in the paraumbilical region but on occasion in the right lower quadrant. The pain usually is out of proportion to the physical findings, with the abdomen being soft or only slightly tender. Often bowel sounds can be heard. Patients commonly develop nausea, with vomiting or diarrhea. In the early stages, diarrhea may test heme-positive but usually is not grossly bloody.

The clinical history is often suggestive of the etiology of the embolus. Classically, patients have stigmata of cardiac disease, namely atrial fibrillation, recent myocardial infarction, or rheumatic valvular disease. Obtaining a careful history often reveals that the patient has had prior episodes of embolization, either in the form of stroke or peripheral arterial emboli. Angiography usually demonstrates that the origin of SMA is patent; the embolus forms a filling defect, with a meniscus sign located 6 to 8 cm distally, allowing perfusion of the proximal two to three jejunal branches. The more distal jejunal and the ileal and colic branches do not opacify.

Treatment. A variety of nonoperative treatments have been suggested and on occasion are successful. Intra-arterial instillation of papaverine, generally via the angiographic catheter that has been left in place, is often helpful. Likewise, there are case reports of patients who have developed spontaneous resolution of their symptoms after volume resuscitation and, on occasion, the administration of dextran.

Although nonoperative treatment is occasionally successful, the patient's best chance of survival is with surgical treatment. A celiotomy is performed. Usually, a transverse arteriotomy is performed in the SMA as it emerges beneath the pancreas. Following embolectomy and restitution of arterial flow, the intestine is examined for viability. A variety of tests have been proposed to aid in the detection of irreversibly ischemic intestine. In general, clinical observation is usually sufficient. The intestine is examined and is allowed to be perfused for about 30 minutes while covered with warm laparotomy sponges. Obviously, necrotic intestine is resected, the cut ends are stapled, and the patient is returned to an intensive care unit. In general, the patient is returned to the operating room 24 hours later to examine the marginally ischemic areas of bowel. Following this second-look procedure, anastomosis can be performed in areas of viable intestine.

The causes of the high mortality associated with mesenteric artery embolectomy are several. Patients often have advanced cardiovascular disease and are unable to tolerate a major operative procedure. The diagnosis of mesenteric artery embolization may be delayed, resulting in more extensive necrotic bowel. Systemic sepsis, as well as the long-term problem of having insufficient intestine remaining to maintain health, also contribute to mortality.

Acute Mesenteric Artery Thrombosis

Acute mesenteric arterial ischemia is most commonly due to an orificial disease of the SMA, usually an extension of midaortic occlusive disease into the orifice of the SMA. Usually it has been a long time developing and is associated with concomitant orificial disease of the celiac artery and IMA. Patients commonly give a history suggestive of the development of mesenteric ischemia. Symptoms include weight loss, postprandial pain, and altered bowel habits. Acute abdominal findings generally are indicative of intestinal necrosis and appear late in the evaluation of the disease. Angiography is the definitive diagnostic tool. Both anterior-posterior and lateral angiograms must be obtained so that the origin and proximal 5 to 6 cm of the SMA, celiac artery, and IMA can all be evaluated. Because of the abundant collateral circulation, several levels of occlusive disease are usually seen. It is unusual for patients to develop mesenteric ischemia if two of the three mesenteric arteries are not markedly diseased or occluded. Evidence of collateral circulation is often seen, namely a wandering mesenteric collateral or prominent marginal artery of Drummond.

Surgical Treatment. Surgical correction is the only effective means of treatment. The surgical procedure depends on the anatomy of the occlusive disease. In general, revascularization of a number of vessels is recommended. When disease of both the celiac artery and SMA are present, the author prefers to bypass both these lesions. The arteriotomy is usually made in the aorta, just proximal to the origin of the celiac axis, and is extended into the celiac artery beyond the distal extent of disease. The proximal anastomosis is constructed so as to patch open the celiac obstruction. The graft is then anastomosed distally to the SMA, usually just distal to the pancreas. Using this technique, both mesenteric vessels can be revascularized using just two anastomoses. Alternatively, grafts can also be based on the infrarenal aorta. The celiac circulation is bypassed with a graft to the hepatic artery, and the SMA is bypassed to that portion of the artery distal to the pancreas. Often, because of the coexistence of aortic occlusive disease, the surgeon must be innovative in revascularization. Following revascularization, the intestine is examined much the way it is in mesenteric embolization; obviously necrotic intestine is removed; marginal intestine usually is left to be evaluated after 24 hours by a second-look operation. If the diagnosis and the therapy are instituted before irreversible intestinal changes occur, the intestine will totally "pink up" and preclude the necessity for a second-look operation.

Nonocclusive Mesenteric Infarction

Nonocclusive mesenteric infarction is a secondary problem of shock, most commonly cardiogenic shock secondary to myocardial infarction, massive congestive heart failure, or sepsis. The intestine responds to hypotension and low cardiac output by intense vasoconstriction: if the hypotension persists, irreversible changes in the intestine can occur. Vasoconstriction results from alpha-adrenergic stimulation, release of vasopressin or of renin-angiotensin, or administration of digitalis. When prolonged, it becomes irreversible. Because the intestinal ischemia is secondary to another life-threatening illness, therapy has been associated with high mortality rates. Angiographic findings in this disease include spasm of segmental branches of the SMA, which can be either diffuse or focal. If the condition is diagnosed relatively early, injection of vasodilating agents into the SMA via an arterial catheter is possible. Agents such as papaverine and tolazoline can be tried. Digitalis should be avoided, since it can initiate mesenteric vasoconstriction. Patient care should be vigilant. Surgical intervention is only indicated if the patient develops signs of an acute abdomen as a result of intestinal necrosis.

Mesenteric Venous Thrombosis
Mesenteric venous thrombosis is often seen in the course of coagulopathy, the result of a clotting abnormality such as heparin-induced platelet aggregation, or in protein-C, protein-S, and antithrombin III deficiencies. The clinical history often reveals previous episodes of thrombophlebitis involving the lower extremities. The diagnosis can be made with contrast-enhanced CT examination. Symptoms consist of the insidious onset of vague abdominal pain, abdominal distention, change in bowel habits, nausea, and occasionally mild fever. Bowel sounds are often hypoactive. Angiography will often include findings of reflux of contrast into the aorta because of spasm of the SMA, prolongation of the arterial phase, and intense opacification of thickened intestinal wall. Intravenous heparin administration is the preferred treatment, with intervening surgical therapy for complications of intestinal ischemia.

SUGGESTED READING

Bergan JJ. Visceral ischemia syndromes. In: Moore WS, ed. *Vascular Surgery: A Comprehensive Review.* Philadelphia, Pa: WB Saunders Co; 1991.

Bulkley GB, Hoglund UH, Morris JB. Mesenteric blood flow and the pathophysiology of intestinal ischemia. In: Bergan JJ, Yao JST, eds. *Vascular Surgical Emergencies.* Orlando, Fla: Grune & Stratton; 1987.

Lewis P, Wolfe JHN. Acute mesenteric ischemia. In: Greenhalgh RM, Hollier LH, eds. *Emergency Vascular Surgery.* Philadelphia, Pa: WB Saunders Co; 1992.

Pearce WH, Bergan JJ. Acute intestinal ischemia. In: Rutherford I, ed. *Vascular Surgery.* 3rd ed. Philadelphia, Pa: WB Saunders Co; 1989.

CHAPTER 12

■

Assessment of Abdominal Trauma

John Fildes, MD, FACS

Evaluating the abdomen of an injured patient is a unique clinical challenge. Trauma patients require rapid assessment and urgent decision making based on careful history, physical examination, and few diagnostic tests. The objective of abdominal evaluation is to identify patients requiring emergent exploratory laparotomy. This is in sharp contrast to other surgical patients in whom an organ-specific diagnosis is sought. These surgical patients usually have characteristic history and physical findings that suggest the etiology and location of the abdominal pain complaint. Trauma, on the other hand, produces random and unpredictable injuries that cause significant mortality and morbidity if undetected. Many trauma patients are unable to provide an adequate history. Their physical examinations can be unreliable, equivocal, or interrupted by the need for diagnostic studies or surgical procedures in the head, chest, or extremities. It is of paramount importance to have a clear understanding and algorithmic approach to the abdominal assessment of injured patients.

To simplify this difficult task, there are certain anatomic concepts that are useful in the assessment of abdominal trauma. The only skeletal protection is provided by the lower rib cage superiorly, the vertebral column posteriorly, and the pelvis inferiorly. Fractures of these structures indicate that significant kinetic energy has been applied to the torso and should alert the examiner to the likelihood of intra-abdominal injuries. The *abdomen* lies beneath the diaphragm and above the pelvic floor. Since the diaphragm is mobile and reaches the level of the fourth intercostal space during exhalation, all injuries below the fourth intercostal space are considered abdominal injuries. The *thoracoabdominal region* (Fig. 34) encircles the torso and corresponds to the surface anatomy of the intrathoracic portion of the abdominal cavity. On the anterior torso, it is bounded superiorly by the fourth intercostal space and

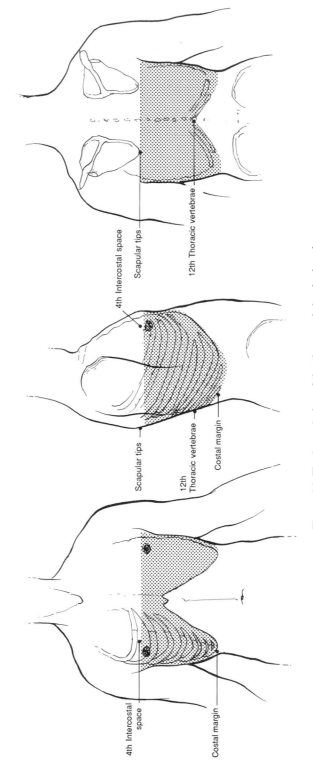

Figure 34. The boundaries of the thoracoabdominal region.

4th Intercostal space

Scapular tips

12th Thoracic vertebrae

Scapular tips

12th Thoracic vertebrae

Costal margin

4th Intercostal space

Costal margin

inferiorly by the costal margin. Its posterior boundaries are the tips of scapulae superiorly and the 12th thoracic vertebra inferiorly. The diaphragm, liver, and spleen are the primary contents of the thoracoabdominal region. The *anterior abdomen* (Fig. 35) is bounded superiorly by the costal margin, laterally by the midaxillary line, and inferiorly by the inguinal ligaments and pubic crest. Its only protection is the soft tissue of the abdominal wall. The *peritoneum* (Fig. 36) is the serosal cavity that lines the abdomen. The organs of the alimentary tract reside in the peritoneal cavity. The *lesser sac* is an extension of the peritoneal cavity and has limited communication with the free peritoneal space. The pancreas, duodenum, and posterior stomach are the primary contents of the lesser sac. The *retroperitoneum* is the space bounded anteriorly by the peritoneal cavity and posteriorly by the vertebral column and paraspinous muscles. It contains the organs of the genitourinary tract, the aorta, and vena cava. The *back and flank region* (Fig. 37) corresponds to the surface anatomy of the retroperitoneum. It is bounded superiorly by the scapular tips, laterally by the midaxillary lines, and inferiorly by the crest of the iliac wings. The *pelvic region* (Fig. 38) encircles the lower torso and corresponds to the intrapelvic extension of the abdominal cavity as well as the pelvic outlet tracts. On the anterior torso it is bounded superiorly by the pubic crest and inferiorly by the perineum and upper thighs. Its posterior boundaries are the crest of the iliac wings superiorly and the gluteal folds inferiorly. The contents of the pelvic region differ in male and female patients. The male pelvis (Fig. 39) contains the most inferior extension of the peritoneum, colon, and bladder. The pelvic outlet tracts in the male are the rectum and urethra. The female pelvis (Fig. 40) contains the same structures and, in addition, the ovaries and uterus. The pelvic outlet tracts in the female are the rectum, vagina, and urethra.

The use of these anatomic regions will greatly simplify the assessment of injuries and need for surgical intervention. These anatomic regions will be used in subsequent sections on blunt and penetrating abdominal trauma to describe a logical and algorithmic evaluation process.

CLINICAL ASSESSMENT

The clinical assessment of an injured patient must combine the art and science of surgical practice. Injury can produce a wide variety of findings that are random and unpredictable. Since the goal of abdominal trauma assessment is to identify patients requiring surgical intervention, the history, physical examination, and ancillary diagnostic studies form the foundation of decision making.

The history begins with information provided by prehospital personnel. Many times the patient is incapable of providing the details of the injury event. It is important to know the mechanism of injury, ie, was it blunt or pen-

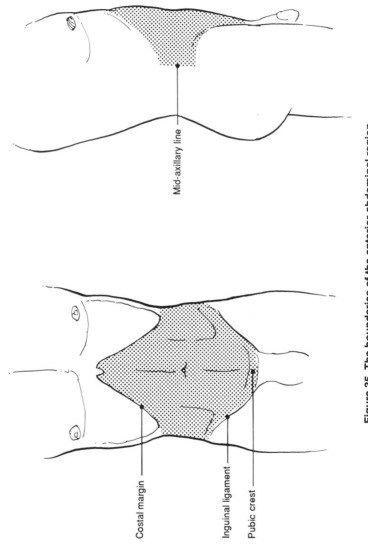

Mid-axillary line

Costal margin

Inguinal ligament

Pubic crest

Figure 35. The boundaries of the anterior abdominal region.

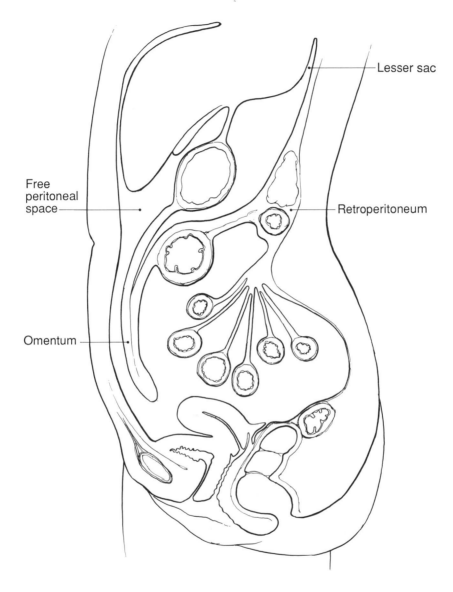

Figure 36. Sagital view and relationship of the peritoneal cavity, lesser sac, and retroperitoneum.

etrating. In the case of blunt injuries the prehospital personnel can describe the scene. If a motor vehicle was involved, it is important to know if the patient was restrained, if the patient was found inside or outside the vehicle, if the vehicle was involved in a frontal or side impact, if there was deformity of the steering wheel or passenger compartment. Penetrating trauma is less am-

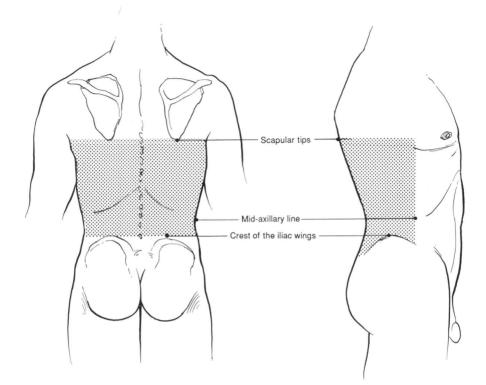

Figure 37. The boundaries of the back and flank region.

biguous and seldom requires prehospital information to assess the abdomen. When patients are awake and alert, they can describe the location and severity of abdominal injury. Descriptions of the size of the knife or gun are generally unreliable and should not be significantly weighed in the history.

The physical examination is extremely important. Inspection comes first. Patients should be completely undressed and examined on the front, back, and sides. The inspection is begun by identifying all injuries and recording them for the permanent record. The examiner should look, listen, and feel all injured areas. Signs of peritonitis, shock, evisceration, and intraperitoneal bleeding should be sought.

Auscultation should be performed in all four quadrants of the abdomen. Since the injuries may be evolving during the first examination, it is important to note the location of diminished bowel sounds and abnormal auscultatory findings such as "crunching" caused by rib fractures and subcutaneous air, bowel sounds in abnormal areas such as the lower chest, and bruits. Aus-

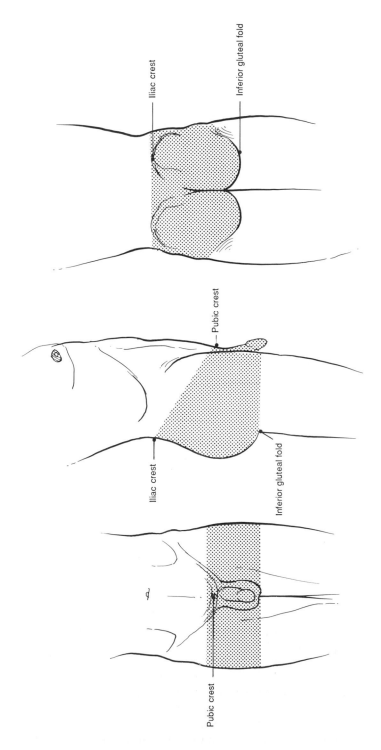

Figure 38. The boundaries of the pelvic region.

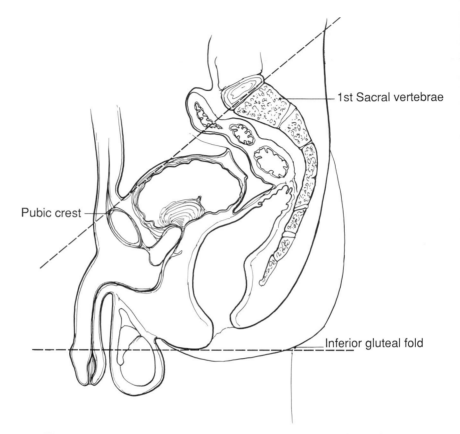

1st Sacral vertebrae

Pubic crest

Inferior gluteal fold

Figure 39. The anatomic boundaries and contents of the male pelvis.

cultation should be performed before palpation to minimize stimulation of the gastrointestinal viscera and subsequent false-positive findings.

Palpation must be carefully performed. Abrasions, contusions, rib fractures, and pelvic fractures may be present. These can create distracting pain for the patient and cause equivocal findings. Evidence of peritoneal irritation can sometimes be demonstrated by shaking the gurney with the knee without touching the abdomen. If the patient experiences pain and demonstrates guarding, peritonitis is present. Having the patient cough or raise the shoulders from the gurney will accomplish the same objective. Start palpating the abdomen away from the injury site and look for signs of voluntary and involuntary guarding. Rigidity, rebound tenderness, and referred tenderness are strong signs of peritonitis. It is important to note that 30% of patients with

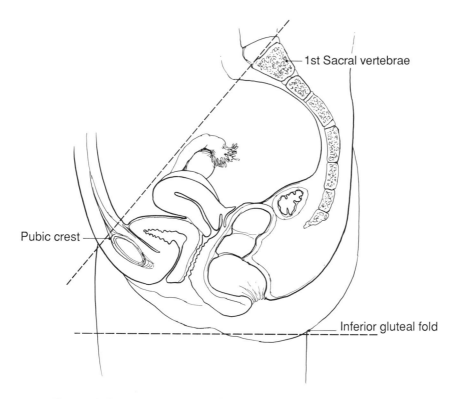

Figure 40. The anatomic boundaries and contents of the female pelvis.

blood in the peritoneum on initial examination will not have peritonitis. Blood becomes a peritoneal irritant after 1 hour of exposure.

The role of diagnostic studies is limited at this point in the clinical evaluation. The most common studies performed are roentgenograms, complete blood cell counts (CBC), and serum chemistries. The role of peritoneal lavage and computed tomography will be described below. Roentgenograms of the cervical spine, chest, and pelvis are usually the first to be available. Alterations in the spinal roentgenograms should indicate the likelihood of altered pain sensation below the level of the injury. In this case, the physical examination is of limited use. The chest roentgenogram may reveal free air below the diaphragm or herniation of abdominal viscera into the chest. Fracture of the lower ribs often suggests injury to the liver or spleen. Hematomas will displace the gastrointestinal gas patterns away from the site of injury. Pelvic fractures are frequently associated with other intra-abdominal injuries, especially the urinary tract. Laboratory analyses like the CBC are nonspecific.

While they may indicate a falling hematocrit, they will not identify the body cavity where there is bleeding. White blood cell counts are not elevated early in the course of evaluation because systemic responses to peritoneal irritation have not had time to be established. Other tests such as amylase or liver enzyme studies follow this same pattern and are not useful.

Although the history and physical examination are the most accurate and sensitive indicators of intra-abdominal injury in the fully awake and alert patient, many patients will not fit into this category. Patients who have evaluations that are equivocal, unreliable, or those who are not accessible for serial abdominal examinations are candidates for an ancillary diagnostic study.

BLUNT ABDOMINAL TRAUMA

Blunt abdominal trauma is a common problem in injured patients. After the airway, breathing, and circulation have been managed, the abdominal assessment is performed. Since the objective is to identify patients requiring surgical intervention, it is important to look for the absolute indications for emergent exploratory laparotomy. They include persistent or recurring shock, peritonitis, and injury to the gastrointestinal tract. Gastrointestinal tract injury is indicated by bleeding from the nasogastric tube or rectum, as well as the presence of free air in the peritoneum or retroperitoneum on initial roentgenographic studies. Patients having one or more of these findings do not require additional diagnostic tests but should undergo emergent exploratory laparotomy.

The difficulty arises when these findings are not immediately present. This group of patients typically have an unreliable or equivocal physical examination or will not be available for serial examination. Unreliable physical examinations are caused by closed head trauma, spinal cord injuries, substance abuse, distracting pain from fractures or other major injuries, and inappropriate behavior. Equivocal physical examinations are caused by contusions and abrasions to the abdominal wall, lower-rib fractures, pelvic fractures, or abdominal pain that is difficult to differentiate from peritonitis. Patients who are awake and alert will frequently not be available for serial abdominal examinations if they require general anesthesia for other injury repairs or are being transferred to other facilities. When any of these situations is present, the intra-abdominal contents must be assessed using ancillary diagnostic studies. The two most popular studies are the peritoneal lavage and the computed tomography (CT) of the abdomen. While each of these studies has advantages and disadvantages, they share a diagnostic accuracy of greater than 95%. Peritoneal lavage is inexpensive and can be rapidly and easily performed. The procedure consists of inserting a lavage catheter into the peritoneum through a small infraumbilical midline incision (the open technique) or by needle puncture of the peritoneum and passage of guide wire for lavage catheter placement (the closed technique). The complication rate for each of these techniques is less than 1%. One liter of intravenous fluid is introduced and allowed to mix in all four quadrants of the peritoneum. The fluid is drained and sent for analysis. A positive lavage is indicated by less than 100 000 red blood cells (RBC) per cubic centimeter, less than 500 white blood cells (WBC) per cubic centimeter, or the presence of intraluminal material like bile, bacteria, or feces. Its major limitations are inability to evaluate retroperitoneum, lesser sac, and subcapsular solid organ injuries. CT produces high resolution radiographs, which allow evaluation of these areas. It is useful when nonoperative management is planned, especially in children. Injuries to specific solid organs can be identified and graded by severity. Other positive findings include free blood in the peritoneum, hematoma formation, and extravasation of contrast from the gastrointestinal or urinary system. Its major disadvantages are expense, need for an experienced radiology team, and difficulty in diagnosing hollow viscus injury.

The most common organs injured in blunt abdominal trauma are spleen 25%, liver 15%, and kidney 12%. It is important to appreciate that hollow viscus injury is present in 10% of cases.

PENETRATING ABDOMINAL TRAUMA

Penetrating abdominal trauma is caused by gunshot wounds, stab wounds, and other objects that enter the torso. After the airway, breathing, and circulation have been managed, the abdominal assessment is performed. The decision to perform an exploratory laparotomy follows a logical order, based on the likelihood of internal injuries requiring surgical repair. Patients with persistent or recurring shock, peritonitis, bleeding from the nasogastric tube or rectum, free air in the peritoneum or retroperitoneum, evisceration, or retained stabbing implement require emergent exploratory laparotomy. An abdominal roentgenogram with intravenous contrast (IVP) is rapidly performed. This "one-shot IVP" is used to demonstrate two functioning kidneys. It is not intended to identify renal injuries but rather to establish the presence of a functioning kidney on the uninjured side should nephrectomy be necessary.

The management of gunshot wounds is reasonably straightforward. Stab wounds, however, can be more difficult to evaluate. These two types of penetrating injuries will be discussed separately.

Gunshot wounds entering the torso from the thorax to the thighs can penetrate the abdomen. Of gunshot wounds that penetrate the abdomen, 98% will produce internal injuries requiring surgical repair. Therefore, all gunshot wounds that penetrate the abdomen require exploratory laparotomy. Occasionally, abdominal penetration is equivocal. This occurs primarily with tangential gunshot wounds to the torso. A peritoneal lavage count of less than 10 000 RBCs/cc indicates peritoneal penetration, and an exploratory laparotomy is performed. Gunshot wounds in the thoracoabdominal area, back and flank and pelvis, with equivocal abdominal penetration are less common. These unique gunshot wounds can be evaluated like stab wounds.

Stab wounds to the anterior abdomen can be managed in several ways. It is important to realize that only 50% of stab wounds penetrate the peritoneum and only 50% of these produce injuries requiring surgical repair. Our approach is to identify patients with indications for emergency exploratory laparotomy. These patients are rapidly prepared for surgery. Stable patients who are awake and alert can be evaluated with serial abdominal examinations. If they develop shock or peritonitis they are explored. All others are discharged after 24 to 48 hours of observation. Patients who cannot be reliably evaluated with serial abdominal examinations pose a unique challenge. Peritoneal lavage, local wound exploration, laparoscopy, and mandatory exploratory laparotomy have been advocated. Of these diagnostic tests, we have found peritoneal lavage to be reliable in predicting the need for exploration.

There are three types of stab wounds that are difficult to evaluate. They are categorized as thoracoabdominal wounds, back and flank wounds, and pelvic wounds. Thoracoabdominal wounds may enter the thorax, penetrate the diaphragm, and injure the intra-abdominal contents. Evidence of peritoneal penetration provokes exploratory laparotomy in these patients. We use a peritoneal lavage count of greater than 10 000 RBCs/cc to demonstrate peritoneal penetration. A chest tube is placed in the injured hemithorax and an exploratory laparotomy is performed to repair the diaphragm and all intra-abdominal injuries. Back and flank wounds can cause retroperitoneal injuries as well as penetration of the peritoneum. Injuries to the retroperitoneal portions of the duodenum and colon are particularly dangerous. We use a peritoneal lavage count of greater than 10 000 RBCs/cc to demonstrate peritoneal penetration. An exploratory laparotomy is performed to repair all injuries in the peritoneum and retroperitoneum. If the peritoneal lavage count is less than 10 000 RBCs/cc, a CT scan with intravenous, duodenal, and colonic contrast is performed. This "triple contrast CT" delineates retroperitoneal injury with a diagnostic accuracy greater than 95%. Pelvic wounds can cause injuries to the gastrointestinal tract, genitourinary tract, and gynecologic tract structures in the pelvic outlet as well as penetration of the peritoneum. We use a peritoneal lavage count of greater than 10 000 RBCs/cc to demonstrate peritoneal penetration. In addition, *all* patients receive a pelvic outlet tract diagnostic evaluation consisting of rigid proctosigmoidoscopy, cysto-urethrogram, and vaginal speculum examination. If the lavage count is greater than 10 000 RBCs/cc or the pelvic outlet tract evaluation is positive, an exploratory laparotomy is performed. All other patients are observed.

The most common solid organs injured by penetrating trauma are liver 37%, spleen 7%, and kidney 5%. As a group, however, hollow viscus injuries are more common. The hollow viscus injuries caused by penetrating trauma are small bowel 26%, stomach 19%, and colon 16.5%.

SUMMARY

The objective of abdominal trauma assessment is to identify patients requiring emergent exploratory laparotomy. This is a difficult task because of the random and unpredictable injuries caused by trauma. The history and physical examination are the most accurate tools in the evaluation of patients who are awake and alert. Many patients, however, have findings that are unreliable, equivocal, or the patients are not accessible for serial examination. These patients require ancillary diagnostic studies such as the peritoneal lavage or CT.

Patients with blunt or penetrating abdominal trauma require emergent exploratory laparotomy if any of the following are present:

- Persistent or recurring shock
- Peritonitis
- Bleeding from the nasogastric tube or rectum
- Free air in the peritoneum or retroperitoneum
- Extravasation of contrast material
- Retained stabbing implements
- Evisceration
- Gunshot wounds penetrating the abdominal cavity
- Positive peritoneal lavage or CT

Penetrating wounds that are difficult to evaluate include those of the thoracoabdominal region, back and flank region, pelvic region, or tangential wounds. We perform exploratory laparotomy on all patients with the following findings:

- Thoracoabdominal wounds: peritoneal lavage greater than 10 000 RBCs/cc
- Back and flank wounds: peritoneal lavage greater than 10 000 RBCs/cc *or* positive triple-contrast CT
- Pelvic wounds: peritoneal lavage greater than 10 000 RBCs/cc *or* positive pelvic outlet tract diagnostic evaluation
- Tangential wounds: peritoneal lavage greater than 10 000 RBCs/cc

All patients with significant abdominal trauma who do not meet the above criteria for exploratory laparotomy should be observed with serial examination for 24 hours to rule out missed injuries.

SUGGESTED READING

Holcroft JW, Blaisdell FW. Trauma to the torso. In: Wilmore DW, Brennan MF, Harken AH, eds. *Care of the Surgical Patient.* New York, NY: Scientific American Inc; 1993.

Trunkey DD. Torso trauma. In: Ravitch MM, Stelchen FM, eds. *Current Problems in Surgery.* Chicago, Ill: Year Book Medical Publishers Inc; 1987.

Trunkey DD, Hill AC, Schecter WP. Abdominal trauma and indications for celiotomy. In: Moore EE, Mattox KL, Feliciano DV, eds. *Trauma.* 2nd ed. Norwalk, Conn: Appleton & Lange; 1991.

CHAPTER 13

■

Abdominal Pain in Children

Janet Meller, MD

The diagnosis of abdominal pain in the pediatric patient can be one of the most challenging aspects of medical practice, for here it is true that children are not just small adults. An infant cannot communicate his symptoms with words, and the medical conditions responsible for abdominal pain in infants and children can be quite different from those of adults. Nevertheless, although history and physical examination are more difficult in the child, the savvy medical practitioner can overcome these obstacles.

Historically, it has been believed that infants do not experience pain; however, it is clear from several studies and our experience that even the tiniest premature infants have pain and, in fact, can manifest their pain in much the same way as older individuals.

PHYSICAL EXAMINATION

In approaching any individual, especially a child, it is important to gain his or her confidence. Infants and children tend to be extremely wary of strangers; moreover, by the age of 6 months, most infants associate physicians with pain. Therefore, it is important to engage the child in a nonthreatening manner before beginning any physical contact.

First, notice how the child is lying and how he interacts with his mother. From infancy onward, the child with peritonitis will lie extremely still, as movement results in pain. These patients may appear lethargic and whimper if disturbed. As a result, spinal taps are often performed in such patients because it may be difficult to distinguish these symptoms from those of spinal meningitis. Lusty cries may be lacking in the severely ill infant. The mother may complain that the child has been more irritable, unable to find a comfortable position, unable or unwilling to suckle, and waking frequently.

During the initial part of the interaction with the child, it is important to defer any invasive procedures until after the examination of the abdomen. Any "needle sticks" will immediately alter the patient's responses. Sitting down on the bed or near the bed will make the examiner less imposing. An older child can be engaged in conversation and some history elicited. Even preschoolers can often pinpoint the location of their "worst pain."

Before actual palpation of the abdomen, it is important to notice if there are any apparent bulges or masses. Auscultation of the abdomen should then be attempted, although in a frightened child this may be difficult. Occasionally it is possible to use the pressure of the stethoscope bell against the abdominal wall to gauge the extent of abdominal tenderness. If the child is sleeping, it is a good opportunity to gently palpate the abdomen. The child with peritoneal irritation will react to gentle palpation even in sleep.

Palpation of the abdomen in the awake child should begin with the part farthest from the site of "worst pain." It is often beneficial to distract the child with idle conversation before touching him or her. Sometimes, one might use the child's own hand or the mother's to palpate the abdomen. At all times it is important to notice the child's facial expressions and to be aware of changes in heart rate or respiratory rate.

Premature infants may react to abdominal pain by crying or grimacing or they may simply become bradycardic or apneic. If they are on continuous oxygen saturation monitoring, a drop in oxygen saturation may also be noticed during painful stimulation. Peritoneal signs such as involuntary guarding can be appreciated even in 700-gram infants.

CONDITIONS CAUSING ABDOMINAL PAIN

Although the physical signs may be present in any age group, the pathologic conditions leading to abdominal pain in infants may be different from those of the older patient and can be discussed separately.

In Neonates

Necrotizing Enterocolitis. The most common indication for emergency surgery in the neonate is an "iatrogenic" one, necrotizing enterocolitis (NEC). In other words, NEC commonly exists as a result of modern medical practice. NEC was not commonly reported until long-term survival of very-low-birthweight and premature infants became commonplace, and clustering of cases within neonatal nurseries has been reported. The pathophysiology of this condition has been linked to a combination of factors: presence of substrate in the intestinal lumen (usually formula), circulatory compromise (eg, hypotensive episode), and bacterial invasion. Immunocompromise has also been implicated. NEC results in a full-thickness loss of integrity of the intestinal wall. It may occur diffusely from stomach to rectum, often with skip areas. Most commonly, however, the disease is confined to the small intestine and colon. It may also present with an isolated perforation, usually of the terminal ileum.

NEC presents with feeding intolerance and bloody diarrhea in a stressed infant, usually a premature or low-birth-weight baby. Rarely, NEC may also occur in full-term infants who present with gastroenteritis or following an operative procedure. The physical examination is characterized by abdominal distention and signs of peritoneal irritation such as involuntary guarding. Often, these patients require endotracheal intubation because of splinting and carbon dioxide retention. Abdominal wall erythema, edema, or discoloration may also be commonly seen where there is gangrenous or perforated intestine.

In general, NEC is managed nonoperatively with nasogastric decompression, parenteral fluids, and parenteral antibiotics. Surgery is indicated when there is progression of disease or failure to respond to medical management. Surgical options include drainage alone for infants weighing less than 1000 grams; however, in general, resection with stoma formation is necessary. An attempt should be made to be conservative when intestine resection is contemplated, as diversion frequently allows bowel that appears severely compromised to recover.

Malrotation. Less common, but of more acute concern, is malrotation with midgut volvulus. The most common reason for surgical consultation in infants and children is vomiting. In the patient with vomiting, it is essential to inquire as to the character of the vomit. The most common *surgical* cause of nonbilious emesis is pyloric stenosis; however, this entity is not usually associated with abdominal pain or obvious physical findings other than a distended stomach and the presence of the pyloric "olive" in the epigastrium. Usually, nonbilious emesis in the infant is related to gastroesophageal reflux and overfeeding. In the neonate with bilious emesis, however, a surgically correctable lesion should always be considered early because a missed midgut volvulus is a life-threatening lesion that, if diagnosed early, can be easily treated.

Aside from bilious emesis, the infant with a midgut volvulus may present with irritability, temperature instability, abdominal distention, and diffuse tenderness, or there may be a paucity of physical findings. Any infant with bilious emesis should have abdominal roentgenograms at the very least, and a barium examination should also be strongly considered. Once the diagnosis of malrotation with or without volvulus is made, emergency surgical intervention is indicated.

Through an upper abdominal transverse incision, the intestine should be delivered and detorsed in a counterclockwise manner. The colon should be completely mobilized, allowing the cecum to be moved to the left side, and the duodenum mobilized, allowing it to lie on the right side. This is the so-called Ladd procedure. An appendectomy is usually performed to obviate any confusion in later life. In the case of compromised intestine, it is important to be conservative, and stomas should be employed rather than primary anastomoses.

Hirschsprung's Disease. Hirschsprung's disease is caused by a deficiency of innervation of the distal intestine, resulting in its failure to empty properly. This causes a functional distal intestinal obstruction. It rarely presents acutely. However, occasionally neonates will present with abdominal distention accompanied by abdominal pain. Usually these infants were initially well; however, they failed to pass meconium in the first 24 hours of life and thereafter became increasingly distended. In such cases, in the absence of peritoneal signs, gentle colonic irrigation with a rectal tube will relieve the distention.

In older patients, the abdominal distention may be accompanied by peritoneal signs related to Hirschsprung's enterocolitis. This entity is related to bacterial overgrowth in the normal intestine and can cause fulminant sepsis. Enterocolitis is generally marked by bloody, foul-smelling diarrhea with crampy abdominal pain. In the absence of peritoneal signs, gentle colonic irrigations with a rectal tube in place accompanied by broad-spectrum antibiotic therapy may be useful. Urgent surgical therapy is indicated.

Enterocolitis may also occur repeatedly in some patients even after definitive treatment for Hirschsprung's disease has been accomplished. These patients present in much the same way, with pain and foul-smelling diarrhea. The reason for this is unclear, although there is some indication that this complication occurs more frequently in patients who have had enterocolitis prior to initial colostomy. Treatment of this is generally conservative, although repeated episodes may indicate a need for revision of the pull-through or, less commonly, permanent colostomy.

In general, in infants with a history of constipation, it is important to question the parents as to the stool pattern in the neonatal period. Failure to pass stool in the first 24 hours is extremely suggestive of Hirschsprung's disease, and a barium enema and rectal biopsy are in order. In older children with a history of chronic constipation, a negative barium enema does not exclude Hirschsprung's disease. If a clinical suspicion exists, a rectal biopsy should be done.

The rectal biopsy may be done using a vaginal punch with some sedation in the clinic. Suction biopsies are used in many institutions; however, because only a scanty amount of tissue is retrieved, the results may be questionable. The gold standard remains a biopsy performed in the operating room. Sufficient muscle must be obtained and it must be at least 1 to 2 cm from the dentate line to be completely accurate. Ideally, permanent sections should be obtained before planning a colostomy. If biopsies are positive, a colostomy should be performed. A seromuscular biopsy is necessary to ensure that the site of colostomy also has ganglion cells.

Definitive treatment for Hirschsprung's disease includes resection of the involved intestine with a pull-through procedure. This is usually done when infants weigh approximately 15 pounds, although primary pull-throughs are now being advocated by some pediatric surgeons.

Meconium Ileus. Meconium ileus is related to cystic fibrosis and caused by inspissated stool within the intestinal loops. Acute symptoms are related to complications of meconium ileus and include volvulus and meconium peritonitis secondary to intestinal perforation. Such patients will present with abdominal distention, peritoneal signs including abdominal wall erythema, respiratory distress, and signs of hypovolemia. After appropriate resuscitation, when perforation is suspected, exploration is indicated. In uncomplicated meconium ileus, conservative measures including repeated Gastrografin enemas and instillation of Mucomyst can be successful.

In Infants

In infants, both volvulus and Hirschsprung's disease may be of concern. The other more common processes that cause abdominal pain and require surgical intervention are intussusception and incarcerated inguinal hernia.

Intussusception. Intussusception classically presents with crampy abdominal pain. Infants may paroxysmally pull their legs up and cry inconsolably. After a short burst of such crying, they may become extremely lethargic. Cramps may be accompanied by bloody stools classically described as "currant jelly stools." Occasionally the patients may have a history of an antecedent upper respiratory infection.

On early physical examination, the abdomen may be soft and nontender. A careful examiner rarely can palpate the "sausage-shaped" mass in the right upper quadrant; however, absence of abdominal signs does not preclude the diagnosis. Later, as the intestine becomes compromised, peritoneal signs may develop.

In the absence of peritoneal signs, given a suggestive history, the next step should be a barium enema. Barium enema will be diagnostic as well as therapeutic, although success in reduction of the intussusception may depend on the expertise of the radiologist. If the barium enema does not demonstrate *free reflux* of barium into the terminal ileum, surgical intervention is necessary. Common reasons for failure of barium reduction include excessive inflammation or intestinal compromise of the intussuscepted intestine or an ileoileal component. In general, however, it is safest to accept a failure of barium reduction, rather than to make dangerous repeated attempts and risk perforation of the intestine.

A right lower quadrant abdominal incision is made and the right colon delivered into the wound. The intussuscepted intestine should be carefully milked out. As lead points are uncommon, it is rarely necessary to open the intestinal lumen. Most surgeons will also perform an appendectomy. In general, plication is unnecessary; however some surgeons prefer to plicate the intestine to prevent recurrence. Recurrences after nonsurgical reduction occur in approximately 12% of patients and in 4% of patients after surgical reduction. A recurrent intussusception after barium reduction in a toddler may be managed by barium reduction once again. Repeated episodes of intussusception, however, may indicate a need for surgical plication. Recurrent intussusception in an older child dictates surgical exploration.

Incarcerated Inguinal Hernia. Incarcerated inguinal hernia is common in infants and can present with abdominal pain. In fact, there is a 12% incidence of incarceration in the first year of life and a much higher incidence of incarceration in premature infants. Often, the mother will not have noticed a previous groin mass. The infant may present with irritability or be off his feed. At the time of diaper change, the caretaker may notice a groin mass.

Early on, the abdomen may be distended and tenderness may only be related to the groin mass. However, in the face of compromised intestine, peritoneal signs may be present. It is appropriate in the absence of peritonitis to attempt manual reduction of the hernia. The maneuver should be similar to squeezing the air out of a balloon rather than trying to reduce the incarceration en masse. If initial attempts fail, sedating medications can help to relax the child enough to reduce the hernia. Less than 85% of acute incarcerated hernias require surgical reduction. It is important to admit any infant who requires sedation to reduce the hernia and operate on the patient semielectively. Any infant with a history of prematurity who is younger than 6 to 9 months of age must undergo apnea monitoring for 24 hours postoperatively.

In Children

Appendicitis. In older children, the most common cause of emergency abdominal surgery is appendicitis. Approximately 20% will be perforated at the time of initial evaluation. This number will be significantly higher in preschool children and in lower socioeconomic groups.

The presentation of appendicitis in older children is similar to that of adults; however, the presentation in preschoolers can be very different. Usually the "classic triad" of right lower quadrant pain, fever, and anorexia is absent.

Preschool children are unable to communicate the early stages of their illness. They may complain of abdominal pain; however, inability to express their symptoms may cause them simply to be irritable. At this point, many children may be misdiagnosed as having otitis media and begun on antibiotics.

As their illness progresses, they may develop vomiting and diarrhea along with the fever. The inability to localize at this point may lead to confusion with gastroenteritis. Any suspicion of possible appendicitis should lead the clinician to admit the patient for observation.

On physical examination, the child may still not be able to localize to the right lower quadrant. However, a careful examiner may be able to appreciate a difference in abdominal wall tone from right to the left side by laying the hand in the midline and pressing down on one side with the thumb and on the other side with the fingers. The abdomen may otherwise be diffusely tender and distended.

Both ultrasonography and barium enema may be helpful in making the diagnosis of appendicitis in the preschool child. It is better to get a diagnostic test early, rather than wait until the child becomes increasingly more toxic. In fact, it may be necessary to use diagnostic tests in preschool children more frequently than in older patients precisely because the history and physical examination may be confusing.

The surgical approach to the child with acute appendicitis includes preoperative fluid resuscitation to a urine specific gravity of 1015 or less and measures to control hyperthermia. Parenteral antibiotics should be used in patients in whom gangrenous or perforated appendicitis is suspected. A Rockey-Davis incision is usually preferable in children, and allows adequate exposure in most cases.

Meckel's Diverticulum. Meckel's diverticulum may also be a source of acute abdominal pain in children. In fact, most cases of symptomatic Meckel's diverticulum occur in childhood. Abdominal pain related to Meckel's diverticulum may occur as a consequence of intussusception or of diverticulitis.

The child with intussusception may present with crampy abdominal pain and evidence of an intestinal obstruction both clinically and radiographically. As this obstruction is generally ileoileal, barium reduction will be unsuccessful.

Meckel's diverticulitis may present with signs and symptoms more typical of acute appendicitis. *It is uncommon to make this diagnosis preoperatively.*

Other Causes of Abdominal Pain in Children. Other causes of abdominal pain may be considered in pediatric patients. Common ones are listed in Table 12. The clinical situation will often help guide the physician; however, to correctly diagnose a nonsurgical cause or a nonintestinal cause, it must be included in the differential diagnosis.

Immunocompromised patients and patients with sickle cell anemia represent an exceptionally difficult diagnostic challenge. It is in this group that a negative laparotomy may be associated with unacceptable morbidity. Radiographic and other diagnostic examinations before surgery are essential in these patients.

TABLE 12. CAUSES OF ABDOMINAL PAIN IN CHILDREN

Ovarian cyst with or without torsion
Constipation
Pelvic inflammatory disease
Primary peritonitis
Diabetic ketoacidosis
Schönlein-Henoch purpura
Sickle-cell anemia
Pancreatitis
Lead poisoning
Enteric infections
Urinary tract infections
Viral infections
"Psychogenic"

Sickle-Cell Disease. Patients with sickle-cell disease frequently present with abdominal pain. It is important to determine whether the patient has a history of abdominal pain crises. These may be recurrent. Patients may have abdominal distention and be diffusely tender on abdominal examination. They usually will not localize to a specific point; however, the pain may be more toward the right side because sludging of sickle cells within the liver may cause tenderness. The patients may even have "peritoneal signs" such as rigidity of the abdominal wall. Objective evidence of intra-abdominal pathology by tests such as barium enema and ultrasonography are necessary before operation in such patients because of uncertainties in physical examination and the risk to the patient posed by negative laparotomy. Often patients will improve after hydration, oxygen therapy, and exchange transfusion.

Schönlein-Henoch Purpura. Schönlein-Henoch purpura is a vasculitis that may be complicated by abdominal pain. The characteristic finding is a rash, with swelling of the extremities and renal involvement. Occasionally, abdominal pain may be the first symptom and be very difficult to distinguish from acute appendicitis. Intussusception may also complicate Schönlein-Henoch purpura. The rash may not appear until 1 week after initial symptoms.

Torsion of the Ovary. Ovarian cysts are not uncommon in young girls. These are frequently dermoid cysts, which can twist when they reach a certain size. The patients will present with acute abdominal pain, often with localization to the right lower quadrant. If the patient does not have obvious peritonitis with localizing signs, ultrasonography may be helpful. If this is discovered at laparotomy, bloody peritoneal fluid may be seen. If a dermoid cyst is seen, the opposite ovary should be bivalved, as bilaterality is not uncommon. If the ovary and tube can be untwisted and they appear viable, an attempt should be made to preserve them. If the pain is due to the cyst alone without a torsion, an attempt should be made to excise the cyst and preserve the ovary and tube. An appendectomy should also be done, especially if a right lower quadrant incision is used.

Pelvic Inflammatory Disease and Pregnancy. Pelvic inflammatory disease (PID) may occur even in patients who are not sexually active. Physical findings include peritonitis with localization in the lower abdomen and may be very similar to appendicitis, although a bilateral component on abdominal examination should be more prominent. In general, patients present with a shorter history and more fulminant course. Pelvic examination may be extremely helpful in such cases.

In any adolescent girl, it is important to elicit the social history in privacy. Patients may be ashamed to admit to being sexually active in front of parents who swear that their children would not engage in sexual activity. Vomiting and abdominal pain may also be a feature of intrauterine or ectopic pregnancy. Pregnancy tests must be obtained in adolescent girls prior to any surgical procedure and should be contemplated in adolescents admitted with abdominal complaints. We have been surprised to discover an unsuspected pregnancy in some girls referred for possible appendicitis.

Psychogenic Abdominal Pain. Abdominal pain is a common complaint among older children and adolescents. In a large, often-quoted study by Apley of 1000 British schoolchildren, abdominal pain of nonorganic origin occurred in 10%. We frequently see children like this in the office or emergency room setting. Their symptoms are generally related to abdominal pain alone. There is rarely an association with vomiting or diarrhea. The pain may be of a chronic nature or may have occurred acutely. In general it is located in the lower abdomen. On physical examination, tenderness and voluntary guarding may be elicited; however, objective signs of inflammation are usually absent.

In this group of patients, a careful social history is necessary. Again, older children should be questioned separately from parents or caretakers. Furthermore, it is important to broach the question of a nonorganic cause very gingerly. On the other hand, diagnostic tests such as barium studies, ultrasonography, and a full metabolic evaluation are also important. A label of nonorganic causes should not be assigned until all possible organic causes, including metabolic and neurologic etiologies, have been excluded. Such causes of pain as abdominal epilepsy have been reported and should be ruled out.

Nevertheless, it is essential to avoid laparotomy in the child with psychogenic abdominal pain because once a laparotomy is performed, the spector of adhesive bowel obstruction looms large. The addition of laparoscopy to the procedures available in the diagnosis and treatment of children with abdominal pain, especially in the group of adolescents with atypical history and physical findings, provides a very important tool, one that can be used instead of the diagnostic laparotomy.

CONCLUSION

The approach to abdominal pain in the child is in many ways similar to that of the adult, although some of the underlying pathologic conditions differ. The key, as always, is careful history, physical examination, and use of diagnostic tests as felt to be indicated by the clinician.

SUGGESTED READING

Apley J. *The Child with Abdominal Pain.* Springfield, Ill: Charles C Thomas Publisher; 1959.

Apley J, Naish N. Recurrent abdominal pain: a field survey of 1,000 school children. *Arch Dis Child.* 1958; 33:165.

Ashcraft KW, Holder TM. *Pediatric Surgery.* Philadelphia, Pa: WB Saunders Co; 1993.

Raffensperger JG, ed. *Swenson's Pediatric Surgery.* New York, NY: Appleton-Century-Crofts; 1980.

Vaughan VC, III, McKay RJ, Nelson WE, eds. *Nelson Textbook of Pediatrics.* Philadelphia, Pa: WB Saunders Co; 1992.

Welch KJ, Randolph JG, Ravitch MM, et al. *Pediatric Surgery.* Chicago, Ill: Year Book Medical Publishers Inc; 1986.

CHAPTER 14

■

Acute Pelvic Pain in Women

Mark Vajaranant

To be adept at evaluating acute or acutely worsening pelvic and lower abdominal pain in reproductive-aged and postmenopausal women a clinician
must have a working knowledge of female pelvic anatomy and how to perform a thorough examination of its components. In addition, the clinician
should have a basic knowledge of the physiology of the menstrual cycle and
the changes that occur in the female genital tract with reproduction and ag-
ing. Before discussion of the individual disorders, a brief review of the history and physical examination as well as the other means of evaluating the
woman with acute pelvic pain is offered. Unfortunately, space limitations and
the goals of this text prevent detailed discussion of these topics as well as the
treatment of the various conditions. Nevertheless, it is hoped that at the com-
pletion of this section clinicians faced with women with acute pelvic pain will
feel comfortable with their ability to evaluate those patients and arrive at a
working diagnosis. For those readers who are interested in deepening their
understanding of the individual disorders it is suggested that they refer to the
list of excellent references at the end of this section for a more comprehensive
review of all these topics.

HISTORY

Obtaining the history from a woman with acute pelvic pain differs from the
evaluation of a man with abdominal pain only in obtaining more information
regarding female-specific issues. The history should initially focus on the pain
itself. The time course and evolution of the pain will give important clues as
to its etiology. For example, rupture of an ovarian cyst will frequently be accompanied by an abrupt onset of severe pain. Torsion of an adnexal structure,
on the other hand, can present with a waxing and waning course, followed
by a sudden worsening. Another important historical clue would be the location of the pain and whether there is radiation or migration of the pain. Pain

that is primarily suprapubic may point to a primary uterine problem or cystitis. Pain that begins in the pelvis and lower abdomen and spreads to the upper abdomen may indicate a spreading peritonitis, whether the cause is infection as with pelvic inflammatory disease or blood from a hemorrhagic pelvic structure. The pain of pelvic pathologic conditions is frequently referred or radiated to the rectum, vagina, lumbosacral region of the back, and the anterior aspects of the thighs because of the innervation and proximity of these structures. Posterior thigh pain is rare with gynecologic disorders and occurs primarily if there is irritation of the sciatic nerve by endometriosis or invasive gynecologic cancers. Shoulder pain is the classic symptom of diaphragmatic irritation, and this should be sought in the history, especially if a developing diffuse peritonitis or intra-abdominal bleeding is suspected. Pain that began in the epigastrium, periumbilical region, or flank may not be gynecologic at all but rather gastrointestinal or renal in origin. Exacerbating and relieving factors are important historical findings also. Pain with movement is more often associated with peritonitis but can also be associated with torsion of adnexal structures or large masses that pull on their pedicle and other pelvic structures. Dyspareunia, especially deep dyspareunia, may indicate pathologic conditions of the ovaries or fallopian tubes, as these structures lie in the pouch of Douglas and are subject to contact with the penis through the vaginal wall during intercourse. The nature and character of the pain may offer some clues as to its etiology and should be characterized. As an example, the pain associated with spontaneous abortion is often described as suprapubic, midline, crampy, and menstrual-like.

Establishing the patient's normal menstrual pattern is extremely helpful in the more common causes of acute pelvic pain, as they are often associated with menstrual aberrations or vaginal bleeding. The occurrence of the pain in relation to the menstrual cycle may provide helpful clues. Pain occurring soon after the start of menses may support a diagnosis of gonococcal pelvic inflammatory disease. The pain that occurs midcycle or in the luteal phase may be due to physiologic cysts of the ovary. The patient's form of contraception is another essential historical point that should be investigated. Hormonal contraception of any kind decreases the risk that the cause of the pain is ovarian disease because of the suppression of follicular cyst formation. Progesterone-only contraceptives, including progesterone-containing intrauterine devices (IUDs), raise the specter of ectopic pregnancy in the woman with a positive pregnancy test. Pregnancy in any IUD user is also more likely to be in an ectopic location. IUD use also raises the risk of infection but only if inserted in the previous 3 months. A previous tubal ligation markedly decreases the risk of pelvic inflammatory disease (PID). The patient's sexual history and past history of sexually transmitted disease and PID should not be neglected, as this will provide an estimate of the patient's risk for recurrent PID or ectopic pregnancy. A history of recent instrumentation or trauma of the genital tract should be actively sought, since the patient will not always actively volunteer this information. Questions regarding sexual history, trauma, and instrumentation should be asked in a matter-of-fact fashion with assurances of confidentiality. As with any good history, associated symptoms need to be sought out. The clinician should ask about fever and chills, gastrointestinal symptoms, urinary tract symptoms, and other concurrent problems.

THE PHYSICAL EXAMINATION

After a thorough history is obtained, the physical examination can be performed. This should begin with an abdominal examination that looks for point tenderness, diffuse tenderness, rebound, the presence and nature of bowel sounds, and other physical signs detailed elsewhere in this text. Only when the abdominal examination is completed should attention be directed to the pelvis. Technically, there are many ways to perform a pelvic examination, and it is assumed that the reader has already been introduced to a particular technique. However, the good clinician adheres to two universal principles of the pelvic examination. First, before performing any of the actual examination, the clinician always tells the patient exactly what is going on and what is going to happen next. The statement "I'm going to touch you now" before the labia majora are separated for insertion of the speculum helps the patient relax, allowing a more accurate and clinically useful examination. Second, regardless of how the examination is actually done, the clinician must use gentle, deliberate movements. This conveys to the patient that the physician is an experienced examiner who appreciates the fact that the pelvic examination is an almost universally unpleasant experience for women. Hurried, jerky, unsure movements are counterproductive; adnexal tenderness can be elicited in any normal woman by the rough and inexperienced examiner! Adhering to these two principles will allow the clinician to obtain more accurate information from the pelvic examination and reduce the incidence of the "false-positive pelvic," in which the pain and discomfort arise not from the disease process but rather from a poorly done physical examination.

Gentle insertion of proper-sized speculum is important. A large speculum may be needed and appropriate for the obese multigravid woman but completely useless in the elderly postmonopausal woman with an atrophic and stenotic introitus. In the latter situation and with pediatric patients, a long-bladed nasal speculum may be more appropriate. The speculum should be inserted its full length before an attempt is made to visualize the cervix. Only once the speculum is inserted its full length should it be slowly withdrawn and manipulated for the cervix to drop into view. If there is excess blood or mucus in the vaginal vault, this should be removed using large rectal swabs. Unless there is profuse bleeding, wadded gauze sponges are inappropriate because of the discomfort they cause. After the cervix is visualized, the four walls of the vagina can be inspected during slow withdrawal of the slightly opened speculum. This allows the walls of the vagina to fall around the tip of the speculum, ensuring a complete view of its entire length. To complete the pelvic examination, a bimanual examination is performed. Well-lubricated index and middle fingers are inserted into the vagina, with the other hand palpating the lower abdomen. Cervical motion tenderness is assessed by trapping the cervix between the two vaginal fingers and moving the cervix from side to side. This puts tension on the peritoneum covering the pelvic organs and if pain is elicited, indicates an inflammation or irritation of this covering. Next, the size, contour, and position of the uterine corpus is determined. Many inexperienced examiners have difficulty assessing the position of the uterus, but it is actually a simple matter. As the fingers are inserted into the vagina, they will first encounter the firm cervix. Upon further entry into the vaginal vault, if the fingers are deflected downward, the uterus can be judged to be retroverted. If not, the uterus is either midposition or anteverted. The adnexa and the cul-de-sac of the pelvis are examined between the pelvic and abdominal hand. An assessment for masses, fullness, and tenderness should be made. Lastly, an essential part of the pelvic examination is the rectovaginal exam. This is important to rule out a rectal mass masquerading as a cul-de-sac or adnexal mass and may be the only way to adequately judge the size of a retroverted uterus. It is also a useful technique for examining patients with a stenotic vagina or intact hymenal membrane.

DIAGNOSIS

Laboratory Tests

The most important test to obtain in all women of reproductive age is a pregnancy test. The only possible exception to this rule are those women who have had a hysterectomy or verifiable bilateral oophorectomy. Regardless of the clinical history of sexual activity or means of contraception, not obtaining a pregnancy test in this group of women is an inexcusable error. The immunoenzymetric technique (a variation of the enzyme-linked immunosorbent assay [ELISA] technique) used in most urine pregnancy tests available in this country is highly sensitive to beta-human chorionic gonadotropin (beta-HCG) and can detect levels as low as 50 mIU/mL. If a woman's urine pregnancy test is negative, provided it used the immuoenzymetric technique, the clinician can feel confident that the woman is not pregnant and a serum quantitative beta-HCG assay need not be obtained. If a woman is pregnant, the serum quantitative value may be of use clinically and should be obtained.

A complete blood count may be of use in evaluating a woman believed to have an infection or concealed hemorrhage. Evaluating the mean corpus-cular volume may assist in determining whether an anemia is an acute or chronic process. A test that may have been overused in the gynecologic patient is the erythrocyte sedimentation rate. The primary problem with this test is its nonspecificity, and it has been shown to be elevated in many pathologic conditions of the female pelvis. Rarely is this test useful in the evaluation of a woman with acute pelvic pain. A quantitative serum progesterone determination is useful when evaluating a woman early in pregnancy and can provide the clinician with valuable information regarding the normalcy of a pregnancy.

Cervical cultures and cervical Gram's stain may be useful in evaluating a woman for infection, but it should be remembered that there is ample evidence that they are unreliable predictors of the type of pelvic infection a woman may have. Cultures are only useful if positive and then for reasons of follow-up care to ensure eradication of the offending organism.

Culdocentesis

Nonclotting blood from culdocentesis provides strong evidence of intra-abdominal bleeding. An 18-guage spinal needle is inserted through the wall of the posterior vaginal fornix into the pouch of Douglas in order to aspirate any fluid that may have collected in this most dependent part of the pelvis. It is essential that the patient not have a retroverted uterus because the spinal needle would simply be inserted into the uterine corpus in this situation. The pouch of Douglas normally contains a small amount of clear, straw-colored fluid, and if infection is present, the fluid may be noted to be turbid or frankly purulent. If blood is obtained, it is essential to let the collected blood stand for several minutes. Blood that has accumulated in the pelvis because of a bleeding abdominal or pelvic structure will not clot because of autolysis.

Ultrasonography

Ultrasonography can be useful in evaluating a pregnant woman in order to assess the location of the pregnancy. It is also useful to evaluate the nature of a pelvic mass detected on a bimanual examination or to detect a large fluid collection in the cul-de-sac. Another situation in which ultrasonography is helpful is when pain prevents an adequate assessment of the pelvic structures. The best images are often obtained with the endovaginal probe because of the proximity of the probe to the pelvic organs. Ultrasonography for all its usefulness, should not be a routinely ordered study.

Diagnostic Laparoscopy

If there is uncertainty about the diagnosis, hospitalization for observation or diagnostic laparoscopy can be considered. Because of concerns about cost and the morbidity and mortality associated with any operative procedure, diagnostic laparoscopy cannot be used without strong justification.

PELVIC DISORDERS THAT CAUSE PAIN

Ectopic Pregnancy

A woman who presents with abdominal pain and a positive pregnancy test should be considered to have an ectopic pregnancy until proven otherwise. Historical risk factors obtained from the patient include a previous history of sexually transmitted disease or PID, as the damage to the fallopian tubes in these conditions predisposes to ectopic implantation. Other risk factors for tubal damage and hence ectopic pregnancy include any sort of pelvic surgery, tubal ligation, previous ectopic pregnancy, and endometriosis. Ovulation induction, possibly because of elevated estrogens, has been associated with an increased risk for ectopic implantation. The use of progesterone-only contraceptives predisposes to ectopic pregnancy, perhaps through hormonal effects on tubal motility. The use of an IUD increases the risk of ectopic pregnancy, and those IUDs that contain progesterone increase the risk even further.

Before rupture of an ectopic pregnancy, the signs and symptoms vary but usually include abdominal pain, a delay in the onset of normal menses and some degree of vaginal bleeding. The pain of an unruptured ectopic pregnancy is highly variable and there is no such thing as a typical history. If rupture has occurred, the patient will usually report a sudden worsening of the pain. The history with rupture or with significant bleeding from the distal end of the tube will reveal symptoms of peritoneal irritation such as shoulder pain or exacerbation of the pain with movement. Syncope is sometimes reported at the time of rupture. Abnormal vaginal bleeding is a common symptom associated with ectopic pregnancy and is more frequently reported as irregular spotting. However, the vaginal bleeding can be heavy and interpreted by the patient as a normal menstrual flow. The history will often reveal that the last normal menstrual period occurred more than 6 weeks prior to presentation.

During the physical examination, vital signs may be noted to be normal, but tachycardia and hypotension may be evident if significant intra-abdominal bleeding has occurred. Almost all patients with an ectopic pregnancy will demonstrate abdominal pain and adnexal tenderness that is more typically unilateral if there is no rupture. More than a third of patients will have a palpable adnexal mass on pelvic examination. Frequently, there is mild uterine enlargement. If rupture has occurred, the elicited pain can be quite severe and there will be signs of diffuse peritoneal irritation. At this point the situation has become emergent, and operative intervention is necessary. In arriving at the correct diagnosis, pelvic ultrasonography is extremely useful but only if it confirms an intrauterine pregnancy or a pregnancy in an ectopic location. Adnexal masses such as corpus luteum cysts can mimic an ectopic pregnancy on the ultrasonogram, so care must be taken in interpreting the finding of an adnexal mass. A difficult situation arises when the patient's physical findings are not particularly revealing and the ultrasonogram does not locate a pregnancy. A quantitative assessment of serum beta-HCG will markedly assist in these situations. If the beta-HCG level is greater than 5000 to 6000 mIU/mL an intrauterine pregnancy should be visualized with abdominal ultrasonography. Many ectopic pregnancies have associated beta-HCG levels that are less than 3000 mIU/mL and in these cases, endovaginal ultrasonography is clearly superior. Most ultrasonographic vaginal probes are able to identify an intrauterine pregnancy when the beta-HCG levels are greater than 1000 to 1500 mIU/mL. If the quantitative beta-HCG is greater than 1500 mIU/mL and no intrauterine pregnancy is identified by vaginal probe ultrasonography, suspicion of an ectopic pregnancy must be very great.

A serum progesterone level may be useful in evaluating patients with a suspected ectopic pregnancy, especially if the quantitative beta-HCG level is less than 1500 mIU/mL. A progesterone level greater than 15 ng/mL is almost invariably associated with a normal intrauterine pregnancy. If the progesterone level is less than 10 ng/mL the pregnancy is abnormal, either an ectopic implantation or an abnormal intrauterine pregnancy. Progesterone levels between these two values are less helpful.

If there is still a question at this point as to whether the pregnancy is intrauterine or ectopic and the patient has no adnexal tenderness, if she has no adnexal masses by examination or ultrasonogram, and she is hemodynamically stable, she may be managed as an outpatient. This can only be done if the patient will be available for frequent follow-up examinations and she understands the importance of returning for immediate evaluation if her symptoms should worsen. If the patient's symptoms are anything but mild or there is adnexal tenderness or mass, she should be observed closely as an inpatient. Serial quantitative beta-HCGs and complete blood counts are obtained, with an approximate doubling of the beta-HCG level every 48 hours in the case of a viable intrauterine pregnancy. During hospitalization, histologic examination of the uterine contents by dilation and curettage can be considered, with the understanding that an intrauterine pregnancy will be disrupted by this procedure. The identification of chorionic villi on histologic examination is diagnostic of an intrauterine pregnancy. Diagnostic laparoscopy can also be considered for these patients, but it should be remembered that there is a small but quantifiable false-negative and false-positive rate of between 2% and 5% with this procedure.

Treatment of an ectopic pregnancy is most often surgical and this may be accomplished through laparotomy or, under certain conditions, through operative laparoscopy. Chemotherapy with methotrexate is an approach that has demonstrated some success and may be appropriate in special situations.

Spontaneous Abortion

Often, the real difficulty is not in differentiating an ectopic pregnancy from a viable intrauterine pregnancy but rather from an abnormal intrauterine pregnancy. Frequently spontaneous abortion will present with the symptoms of ectopic pregnancy, ie, abdominal pain, abnormal vaginal bleeding, and delayed normal menses. These patients may also have adnexal tenderness or masses resulting from a coexisting corpus luteum cyst. They will also be noted to have abnormalities of beta-HCG and progesterone levels. Historical risk factors for spontaneous abortion are not as useful in making the diagnosis as in other gynecologic disorders but may include such things as a history of alcohol use, heavy tobacco use, known uterine anomalies, or fibroid tumors of the uterus. Uncontrolled diabetes has been shown to be associated with an increased risk of abortion. A history of previous abortions may put the patient at risk for recurrent abortion. The pain of spontaneous abortion is often described as midline or suprapubic in location and crampy in nature. The history of pain can be variable and may be nonexistent or very mild in a woman with threatened abortion. It can also be quite severe with the attempted passage of the products of conception. The bleeding pattern likewise is variable and may be a light spotting with a threatened abortion or a profuse hemorrhage in the case of some incomplete abortions. A history of passage of tissue is not diagnostic of a complete or incomplete abortion, though it certainly supports this diagnosis. On occasion a woman with an ectopic pregnancy will expel tissue from the uterus consisting of decidua, known as a "decidual cast," that can only be definitively differentiated from products of conception by histologic examination. On the physical examination, uterine tenderness is almost always elicited. Again, an adnexal mass or tenderness may be noted if a corpus luteum cyst is present.

Abortion can be classified as threatened, inevitable, incomplete, or complete and the differentiation needs to be made, as management differs. With threatened abortion, an intrauterine pregnancy has been demonstrated and vaginal bleeding is present but usually described as light or spotting. The pain, if any, associated with this condition is mild. An inevitable abortion may be diagnosed if the bleeding is heavy or the cervical os is open but the uterine contents have not been expelled. An incomplete abortion is diagnosed when there is partial expulsion of the uterine contents and the cervical os is open. The patient may report having passed tissue per the vagina and the bleeding may be profuse. Severe cramping usually continues as the uterus attempts to expel the remaining contents. The state of the cervical os is useful in differentiating between the various types of abortion and can easily be assessed when doing the bimanual examination when the examining finger easily passes through an open cervical os. This assessment can also be made during the speculum examination when the tip of a ring forceps passes easily through the cervical opening without any resistance. Any pregnant woman with an open cervical os and significant bleeding should most likely be treated surgically with uterine curettage to empty the uterus of its contents, as these women are at significant risk for profuse bleeding and are prone to infection. A complete abortion occurs when the uterus empties itself and the cervix subsequently closes. The patient may report heavy vaginal bleeding and severe pain that markedly improved after the passage of tissue. If the patient is examined immediately after passage of the uterine contents, the cervical os may be noted to be open, but bleeding will be minimal and curettage is not necessary. Complete abortion occurs most frequently before 6 weeks and after 14 weeks gestation. As stated earlier, inevitable and incomplete abortions are managed with uterine curettage. Threatened and complete abortions are managed observantly as long as significant bleeding or infection has not supervened.

Pelvic Inflammatory Disease

PID is very common and accounts for an enormous sum of money spent on health care each year. One author on the subject points out that it is the most common serious infectious disorder among young sexually active women. Moreover, acute PID has three major long-term consequences that add to its toll on the health of women: chronic pelvic pain, infertility, and ectopic pregnancy. Certain historical factors should be considered when considering the diagnosis of PID. Youth, number of sexual partners, a history of previous sexually transmitted disease, and form of contraception can all provide a rough estimate of the risk for sexually transmitted disease and, therefore, the risk for PID. For example, a previous episode of PID increases the risk for a subsequent case of PID. An IUD will increase a woman's risk for PID but only in the first several months after insertion. Instrumentation of the uterus is also a risk factor for PID. Protective factors that reduce a woman's risk for PID include the use of barrier or hormonal contraceptives. A history of previous surgical sterilization also markedly decreases a woman's risk. PID after 12 to 13 weeks of gestation in a pregnant woman is unlikely, as this is when the amnion fuses with the chorion and effectively seals off the peritoneal cavity from the outside world. PID in this setting and that of surgical sterilization can still occur, probably through hematogenous or lymphatic spread of the offending organism.

There is no typical presentation of PID, but there are certain signs and symptoms that are found more frequently. Lower abdominal pain is perhaps the most common presenting complaint. The pain is frequently localized to the lower abdomen and is worsened with movement or sexual activity, reflecting the peritoneal irritation attendant with this disorder. The pain may also be reported to have spread to involve the upper abdomen, and if this occurs in a woman with PID, it may be a worrisome symptom, indicating the development of a diffuse peritonitis or rupture of a tubo-ovarian abscess. Diffuse peritonitis and the subsequent development of sepsis accounts for most of the mortality of PID today. Right upper quadrant pain that is frequently pleuritic in nature, in conjunction with other findings suggestive of PID, may represent Fitz-Hugh-Curtis syndrome. This is a condition in which the pelvic infection has traveled up the right colic gutter to cause a perihepatic inflammation. The pain of PID takes many forms but is usually localized to the lower abdomen and is bilateral. It is often described as having a gradual onset and reported to be dull or crampy in nature. The duration of the pain is usually less than a week but can be more. Abnormal vaginal bleeding is a fairly common symptom and can be heavy but more frequently is described as spotting.

A vaginal discharge is a common complaint among women with PID. Fever and chills are symptoms that are sometimes reported but not as frequently as one might suspect for an infectious disorder.

Physical findings are consistent with irritation of the pelvic peritoneum and include lower abdominal tenderness, localized rebound tenderness, cervical motion tenderness, and adnexal tenderness. Other findings may include fever, an elevated white blood cell (WBC) count, and a tender pelvic mass that represents a tubo-ovarian or cul-de-sac abscess. Useful diagnostic tests include the complete blood count and cervical cultures, after pregnancy has been ruled out with a negative pregnancy test. A Gram's stain of cervical material may be useful if organisms suspicious for the gonococcus are identified. An erythrocyte sedimentation rate, for reasons stated earlier, has little utility in evaluating these patients. Culdocentesis can be useful if frankly purulent material is obtained from the cul-de-sac. Finally, ultrasonography has a role in evaluating the patient who has a pelvic mass or when pain is so severe that an adequate examination of the pelvis cannot be performed.

In the past, gynecologists and others have employed a "classic" triad of findings to diagnose PID, and these findings included fever, cervical motion or adnexal tenderness, and an elevated erythrocyte sedimentation rate. Unfortunately, this triad has been shown to occur in less than a fifth of women with laparoscopically proven PID. Two investigators, Eschenbach and Hager, established certain criteria that may improve our ability to accurately diagnose PID. Direct lower abdominal tenderness, cervical motion tenderness, and adnexal tenderness must all be present. In addition, at least one of the following findings must also be present to fulfill the criteria for the diagnosis of PID: (1) fever greater than 38.0° C; (2) leukocytosis of greater than 10 000; (3) purulent material from the pelvis by culdocentesis or laparoscopy; (4) Gram's stain positive for gram-negative intracellular diplococci; or (5) pelvic mass or inflammatory complex on bimanual examination or ultrasonography. These criteria for the diagnosis of PID attempt to improve the specificity of the clinical diagnosis, but the clinician should be aware that some patients will be treated who do not actually have PID. This is acceptable to reduce the long-term sequelae of PID, which make up so much of the morbidity and mortality associated with the disease.

Treatment of PID in this country is generally accomplished on an outpatient basis. It is imperative that patients who undergo outpatient treatment be reexamined in 48 to 72 hours to assess response to antibiotic therapy. There are certain situations in which hospitalization for treatment should be considered and these include: if there is a question about the diagnosis, if the patient is unable to comply with outpatient therapy and follow-up, and if the patient is nulliparous. If the patient is pregnant, has an IUD, an adnexal complex, or has PID secondary to genital tract instrumentation, she should be hospitalized, as these conditions are all associated with more severe PID or PID that is probably more effectively treated with intravenous antibiotics. In closing the discussion of PID it should be emphasized that in absolute numbers, the mortality of PID is about threefold higher per year than that from ectopic pregnancies! This fact should serve to underscore the seriousness of this disorder.

Torsion of Adnexal Structures

Torsion occurs when an adnexal structure twists upon its pedicle, consequently interrupting the blood supply to the affected organ. The most common pelvic structure affected in this way is an ovary that has been enlarged by a mass that is most frequently benign. Normal ovaries have been known to undergo torsion, but this occurs most frequently in the prepubescent girl. Predisposing factors include any process that causes an enlargement of the ovary, such as the growth of a benign tumor or pharmacologic ovulation induction. Another circumstance in which ovarian torsion is more likely is during pregnancy, perhaps because the enlarging uterus lifts the ovary out of the ovarian fossa. Invasive malignant neoplasms and endometriomas are less frequently associated with ovarian torsion, perhaps because of the fixation of the organ attendant with these processes. The fallopian tube is usually involved in ovarian torsion but can be the primary cause of adnexal torsion if the tube is enlarged by a hydrosalpinx or other pathologic process. Paratubal cysts are structures that are most frequently found near the fimbriated end of the fallopian tube but may be found anywhere along its length. When these cysts arise from mesonephric duct remnants, they are called Morgagnian cysts, but more frequently, they arise from the tube itself. They range in size from a few millimeters to many centimeters in diameter. They are sometimes pedunculated and as such are subject to torsion.

The presenting symptoms of a woman with torsion of an adnexal structure is the abrupt onset of severe abdominal pain secondary to the ischemia and infarction of the affected structure. The pain is usually reported to be greater on one side. Nausea and vomiting frequently accompany the onset of the pain and these symptoms may confuse the diagnosis with gastrointestinal pathologic processes. The symptoms are sometimes reported to have occurred with a positional change. It is not infrequent that the patient will describe pain that was mild to moderate and intermittent for days prior to the acute onset of severe pain. This probably represents the adnexal structure undergoing partial twisting and untwisting prior to the event that completely interrupted the blood supply to the affected organ.

Physical findings reveal localized lower abdominal tenderness that may be accompanied by localized rebound tenderness. A pelvic mass that is exquisitely tender to palpation is frequently noted on bimanual examination. Significant temperature elevation is not common, nor are marked perturbations of other vital signs. An elevated WBC count may be noted and is most likely due to a demargination phenomenon. Diagnosis is greatly aided by the use of pelvic ultrasonography.

Treatment is surgical, and in the case of the ovary in a premenopausal woman, conservative treatment of the ovary is attempted with an untwisting of the pedicle and fixation of the organ after the removal of any mass. It has been feared in the past that such management would release venous thrombi from the ovarian vein into the circulation, leading to pulmonary emboli, but this has not been borne out by clinical experience. If there has been significant vascular compromise to the point where the ovary is no longer viable, it should be removed, as further necrosis will lead to a continuation of the severe pain experienced by the patient.

Rupture of Ovarian Cysts

The most common ovarian cysts are follicular or "functional" cysts and, indeed, are formed in the first half of every normal menstrual cycle. Follicular cysts can, however, persist abnormally to the second half of the cycle and beyond. Another normal physiologic cyst of the ovary is the corpus luteum cyst that sometimes arises from the corpus luteum after midcycle ovulation. Nonphysiologic cysts of the ovary encompass a host of malignant neoplasms and benign conditions such as endometriomas and mature teratomas (dermoid cysts). All these cystic structures may rupture and release their contents into the abdominal cavity.

In obtaining the history from patients suffering from rupture of an ovarian cyst, the degree of pain may be noted to range from very mild to severe generalized abdominal pain. For example, the midcycle ovulatory "rupture" of a follicular cyst gives rise to a mild pain known as Mittelschmerz, whereas the pain associated with a ruptured dermoid cyst may be excruciating. Regardless of the type of cyst that has ruptured, the pain is generally described as having a sudden onset and initially being localized to one side of the lower abdomen. The pain can rapidly spread to involve the entire abdomen. The patient may report that she was engaged in some activity such as sexual intercourse, exercise, or physical labor when symptoms first occurred. The patient may also report some sort of trauma to the pelvis such as a blow to the lower abdomen or even a pelvic examination by a physician immediately prior to the onset of symptoms. A syncopal episode immediately after the onset of the pain is not uncommon and by itself should not be a cause for undue concern. The patient will also report that the pain is worsened with movement, a symptom consistent with the peritoneal irritation common to all symptomatic cysts when ruptured. Some cysts that are large may be associated with reports of a previously existing dull pelvic or back ache or feeling of heaviness and pressure in the pelvis or lower abdomen.

On physical examination, vital signs are typically unrevealing. A mild and stable tachycardia may be the result of the sometimes severe pain associated with cyst rupture. Rising tachycardia, falling blood pressure, or orthostatic changes are all worrisome and may indicate significant intra-abdominal bleeding, which is perhaps more commonly noted with rupture of a corpus luteum cyst. Physical findings are consistent with peritoneal irritation, with abdominal tenderness and rebound tenderness. Cervical motion and bilateral adnexal tenderness may be noted on bimanual examination. An adnexal mass may also be noted. Pelvic ultrasonography may be useful if findings demonstrate an adnexal mass or unusual amount of fluid in the pouch of Douglas. Culdocentesis can be useful if it reveals the nonclotting blood of a bleeding corpus luteum cyst or the thick, chocolate-like substance from a ruptured endometrioma.

Management of a ruptured ovarian cyst depends on the nature of the cyst contents and the severity of the symptoms, with the only caveat being to operate if there is evidence of intra-abdominal bleeding. Rupture of follicular cysts usually causes little if any pain but has been known to cause severe pain with syncope, nausea, and vomiting. Fortunately, significant bleeding with this condition is rare, and symptoms resolve rapidly with nearly complete resolution in 12 to 24 hours. Rupture of a corpus luteum cyst usually occurs in the late luteal phase, is usually accompanied by somewhat more severe symptoms, and notably, brisk bleeding can occur, leading to signs of hemorrhagic shock. Rupture of a dermoid cyst or endometrioma is often accompanied by severe chemical peritonitis, and surgical therapy is warranted if for no other reason than to clean the abdominal cavity and relieve the patient of her pain.

Leiomyomas

Leiomyomas, or uterine fibroids, are a common condition of the uterus, which is most often asymptomatic but may become troublesome, with abnormal uterine bleeding, pressure or obstructive symptoms, recurrent abortions, or pain. This condition may cause acute pain because of carneous degeneration or torsion of a pedunculated myoma. The history is typically unrevealing unless the patient has been diagnosed with uterine fibroids before the onset of acute pain. However, the patient may report symptoms of pelvic heaviness or pressure, enlargement of the lower abdomen, irregular vaginal bleeding, or urinary frequency, resulting from the pressure of the myoma on the bladder. The pain is generally severe but may be reported as a dull ache. It is most often midline and suprapubic in location.

The physical examination reveals an enlarged uterus with an irregular contour. There may be exquisite point tenderness of palpable myomas. The myoma itself may have a soft, spongy feel to it rather than the firm consistency of normal uterine tissue. If the cause of the pain is a pedunculated myoma that has undergone torsion, the signs and symptoms may be those discussed under torsion of adnexal structures. Indeed, it may be difficult to differentiate the two conditions on the basis of history and physical findings. Carneous degeneration most frequently occurs during or after pregnancy. During pregnancy this occurs when the myoma enlarges rapidly under estrogen stimulation and outgrows its blood supply. In the postpartum period acute degeneration can follow a marked decrease in blood flow to the uterus secondary to postpartum involution.

During pregnancy the treatment is generally aimed at control of pain with powerful analgesics. The only exception to this rule is if the myoma is pedunculated on a small pedicle that is easily ligated and transected. If the patient is not pregnant, surgical therapy is often indicated, but occasionally conservative management with analgesics is effective.

Endometritis

Endometritis is an uncommon condition in a woman who was not recently pregnant but may occur transiently in a woman with PID or a woman who has recently undergone some sort of uterine instrumentation. It is an infectious disorder that arises when bacteria that normally inhabit the colon and vagina are able to gain access to the uterine cavity by transcervical migration. Endometritis is most commonly encountered in patients who are within 7 to 10 days of a pregnancy. After this period of time the condition becomes uncommon because by then the cervix has closed and lengthened to the point where it acts as a barrier to the invasion of pathogens.

The patient who develops endometritis will have one of the historical factors mentioned above. She will also frequently report fever and chills. Gastrointestinal symptoms are rare, and a report of vaginal bleeding is not helpful because this is part of the normal puerpereum. A foul-smelling discharge from the vagina is sometimes reported by the patient and noted during the physical examination. The pain is localized to the lower abdomen and may be described as crampy or dull.

Physical findings include an elevated temperature and elevated WBC count. In evaluating the WBC count in someone who was recently pregnant, it is important to realize that there may be marked leukocytosis to as high as 30 000 immediately after delivery, and the count falls gradually over the next few days. Infection should be suspected in the symptomatic patient, however, if the count is greater than 15 000. On abdominal examination there is lower abdominal tenderness, usually noted to be predominantly in the midline. Rebound tenderness is rare unless peritonitis has developed. Uterine tenderness is easily elicited when the uterus is palpated between the vaginal and the abdominal hand. If the infection has spread beyond the uterus, cervical motion and bilateral adnexal tenderness will be marked. At this point there is no difference between endometritis and PID, with both consisting of a pelvic infection and pelvic peritoneal irritation.

Traditionally, treatment of endometritis has involved hospitalization of the patient for intravenous antibiotics because of the microbiologically complex nature of the infection and the frequent involvement of anaerobic bacteria.

Endometriosis

Endometriosis is a disorder in which there is ectopic implantation of endometrial tissue outside the uterus. This disorder infrequently presents as acute pelvic pain and more often is associated with a history of chronic or cyclic pelvic pain. With history alone it is extremely difficult, if not impossible, to arrive at the correct diagnosis. However, a history of cyclic pain of varying nature and intensity occurring in the perimenstrual period in conjunction with certain physical findings can achieve the diagnosis of endometriosis with reasonable accuracy. These physical findings include the discovery of an endometriotic nodule or implant in the vagina, nodularity of the uterosacral ligaments or the cul-de-sac, or fixation of a retroverted uterus in a woman who has no history of conditions that might predispose to pelvic adhesions. The patient may not experience tenderness on examination unless it is around the time of menses. Otherwise, the history and physical findings of endometriosis are of such protean nature that it is extremely difficult to make the diagnosis accurately without the aid of such procedures as laparoscopy. When endometriosis does present as acute pain, it is more frequently the result of the rupture of an ovarian endometrioma. The signs and symptoms of this event have been discussed earlier under rupture of ovarian cysts. The physical examination may reveal the findings of nodularity and uterine fixation described earlier. Torsion of an ovarian endometrioma is a rare event because of the intense scarring and fibrosis of the pelvic organs attendant with severe forms of this disease, often leading to the so called "frozen pelvis."

Trauma

Genital tract trauma is not an infrequent presenting complaint in the acute care setting and usually occurs in the context of sexual assault or instrumentation of the uterus. Lower abdominal pain is a frequent patient complaint. With sexual assault the immediate concern, beyond the emotional trauma suffered by these patients, is to detect vaginal perforation, lacerations, and to control sources of bleeding. Vaginal perforation should be strongly considered in the pediatric patient and the patient assaulted with a foreign object. Abdominal roentgenograms looking for free air under the diaphragm will confirm the diagnosis. Bleeding from lacerations is usually obvious but may be hidden, especially if the delicate vessels of the broad ligament have been torn. Bleeding into the broad ligament may dissect into the retroperitoneum, effectively concealing a large blood loss. On bimanual examination careful palpation of the adnexa and sweeping of the pelvic side wall will reveal an adnexal mass or fullness of the side wall. Ultrasonography, computed tomography (CT), and magnetic resonance imaging (MRI) may markedly assist the clinician in detecting the presence or absence of broad-ligament or retroperitoneal hematoma.

With uterine instrumentation, the concern is not only perforation and hemorrhage but also injury to other abdominal organs. The complications from uterine perforation can be minimal, as in the case of perforation of the fundus with a blunt uterine sound. It can also be catastrophic, as in the case where the uterine artery is torn with a uterine curette. If perforation occurs in the fundal region, significant bleeding is not as common. However, if the perforation was done with a sharp instrument or suction device, the possibility of intestinal injury should be considered. Intestinal perforation is possible but not likely. More likely is that intestine or omentum was caught by the instrument and pulled through the defect in the uterus, effectively strangulating the trapped organ. If perforation occurred laterally, intestinal injury may still occur, but severe hemorrhage from trauma to the uterine artery and adnexal veins is the more feared complication. Usually, laceration of the uterine artery or adnexal vessels is accompanied by profuse vaginal bleeding, but as in the case of sexual assault, the bleeding may be hidden in the broad ligament or retroperitoneal space and this possibility should be ruled out in such patients. Unless signs of hemorrhagic shock or intestinal obstruction are evident, hospitalization and close observation can be used as management. If signs and symptoms suggestive of intra-abdominal bleeding or intestinal obstruction develop, diagnostic laparoscopy, ultrasonography, CT, and MRI are all useful tools to make a rapid and accurate diagnosis.

SUGGESTED READING

Cunningham FG, MacDonald PC, Gant NF. *Williams Obstetrics*. 18th ed. Norwalk, Conn: Appleton and Lange; 1989.

Herbst AL, Mishell DR, Stenchever MA, et al. *Comprehensive Gynecology*. 2nd ed. St. Louis, Mo: Mosby-Year Book Inc; 1992.

Thompson JD, Rock JA. *Te Linde's Operative Gynecology*. 7th ed. Philadelphia, Pa: JB Lippincott Co; 1992.

CHAPTER 15

■

Abdominal Pain in the Immunocompromised Patient

Alfredo J. Fabrega, MD, FRCSC
Pedro A. Rivas, MD
Raymond Pollak, MB, FRCS (Ed) FACS

The number of patients with compromised immune function is rapidly increasing. This unprecedented trend is due to the acquired immunodeficiency syndrome (AIDS) pandemic, the use of immunosuppressive medications to prevent rejection of transplanted organs and to control autoimmune disorders, and finally to the use of cytotoxic chemotherapeutic agents to treat malignant diseases. These patients may suffer from any of the common causes of an acute abdomen and are also afflicted by a series of problems directly related to their underlying illness and immunocompromised state. As such, immunocompromised hosts present a unique clinical challenge to the surgeon, both in terms of diagnosis and of eventual management. What follows is an orderly approach to the acute abdomen in this burgeoning patient subpopulation, together with a discussion of a number of disease entities peculiar to these individuals.

THE HISTORY

It is important to identify the immunocompromised host early. Most of these patients have a mild to moderate degree of immunocompromise and are affected with the usual abdominal problems seen in the general population. Severely immunocompromised patients (Table 13) are more likely to present with unusual problems, many times caused by opportunistic infections that may not require surgical intervention. A history of malignant tumor, previous organ transplantation, intravenous drug abuse, other risk factors for ex-

TABLE 13. IDENTIFICATION OF SEVERELY IMMUNOCOMPROMISED PATIENTS

Disease	Parameter
AIDS	CD4+ cell count <200/mm³
Transplant recipient	Receiving or recently received antilymphocyte antibodies or high-dose steroids for induction-rejection
Cancer	Induction chemotherapy with neutrophil count <1000/mm³

posure to the human immunodeficiency virus (HIV), or the presence of autoimmune or inflammatory bowel diseases should be carefully noted. Previous use of corticosteroids, cytotoxic chemotherapeutic agents, exposure to ionizing irradiation, HIV-specific drugs (dideoxyinosine [DDI], azothymidine), or a history of infection(s) by an opportunistic pathogen (e.g., *Pneumocystis carinii, Mycobacterium,* or *Legionella*) should further alert the examiner. Unlike the situation in patients with an intact immune response, who manifest many of the symptoms and signs discussed throughout this book, immunocompromised hosts rarely provide a classical history because of their blunted immune reactivity and complex medical problems. Indeed, rapid progression from initiation of symptoms to systemic involvement often occurs as a result of inability to localize the inflammatory or infectious process. Thus vague symptoms of fatigue, malaise, anorexia, poorly localized abdominal discomfort, unexplained diarrhea, disorientation and lethargy, or low-grade fever may be the harbingers of a more serious intra-abdominal disease process. The immunocompromised host may also present with symptoms related to complications of comorbid disease states or their treatment, e.g., intestinal obstruction consequent to strictures, in patients with Crohn's disease; fluid retention and weight gain with renal allograft rejection; abdominal pain from pancreatitis or perforating ulcers in patients taking DDI or corticosteroids respectively.

Elderly, malnourished patients and those on dialysis who are anergic may also be considered immunocompromised. These patients are usually afflicted with common causes of an acute abdomen (perforating ulcer, malignant bowel obstruction, cholangitis, diverticulitis, etc) but tend to seek medical attention late in the course of their disease and also present few signs or symptoms. Although many of the concepts discussed in this chapter are applicable to this group of patients, they usually are not susceptible to the myriad of opportunistic infections seen in other severely immunocompromised patients.

THE PHYSICAL EXAMINATION

The degree of host immunosuppression will often affect those clinical signs commonly seen in otherwise "normal" patients with an intra-abdominal inflammatory process. Thus fever may be absent, whereas in the elderly, hypothermia is often indicative of systemic sepsis. Unexplained tachycardia, confusion, and disorientation may be apparent along with hypotension if the process is long-standing or if there has been abrupt withdrawal of corticosteroid therapy. The general physical examination may reveal a cushingoid appearance, evidence of malnutrition, lymphadenopathy, or skin lesions (eg, Kaposi's sarcoma) often associated with comorbid underlying disease states. Examination of the heart and lungs is crucial to exclude disease processes above the diaphragm that might mimic an intra-abdominal catastrophe (eg, lower-lobe pneumonias) and to exclude complications from intercurrent diseases (eg, pericarditis in uremic patients, perhaps with failed renal allografts). Examination of the abdomen may reveal the scars of previous abdominal surgery, and it is important to inspect the inguinal region and genitalia, because incarcerated hernias are as likely to occur in these patients as in the "normal" population. Bowel sounds may be absent, especially if the process is of some duration, and the abdomen might well be distended and tympanitic. Depending on the degree of immunosuppression, abdominal wall tenderness and rigidity with rebound tenderness may be florid or remarkably absent, even in the presence of purulent peritonitis. The presence of discrete mass lesions and organ enlargement may be easily appreciated in some but absent in others, depending on the nature of the underlying disease and degree of abdominal wall rigidity. Rectal examination, supplemented by flexible sigmoidoscopy when available, as well as a complete vaginal and speculum examination in women is crucial to help exclude inflammatory or neoplastic diseases of the anorectum and female generative organs. In many instances, however, the physical findings are often subtle or unhelpful, especially in severely ill and immunocompromised hosts, and the surgeon will have to resort to a variety of other investigations to aid in the diagnosis.

LABORATORY TESTS AND DIAGNOSTIC IMAGINING

Laboratory and a variety of noninvasive and invasive tests may be required to confirm or exclude diagnostic possibilities. However, leukocytosis may not always be evident, especially where chemotherapeutic agents have been used in the past or marrow suppression exists. Studies of serum electrolytes may reveal underlying renal insufficiency or prerenal azotemia, while the blood count may show the presence of a leukemic process. Liver function studies may be deranged or normal, while serum amylase levels may be suggestive of pancreatitis when high or reflect only an inflammatory intra-abdominal process when slightly elevated. Urine examination and analysis may reveal pyuria typical of cystitis or pyelonephritis or be noncontributory. An obstructive series, including an upright chest roentgenogram, may demonstrate intraperitoneal free air or a pattern suggestive of intestinal obstruction or a nonspecific ileus. In addition, pneumonic or other infiltrative disorders of the lung may be evident. When available and necessary, computed tomography (CT) of the abdomen may provide important diagnostic information, as may ultrasonography when appropriate. When the latter noninvasive modalities are unavailable, some have suggested diagnostic peritoneal lavage to establish or exclude the presence of pus, blood, feces, or malignant neoplasia within the abdomen. Finally, appropriate body fluids are cultured for fungi, mycobacteria, viruses, and parasites. Endoscopy (where indicated) should include mucosal biopsy for culture and histology, where specific stains may demonstrate the offending pathogen or disease.

DIFFERENTIAL DIAGNOSIS

The aphorism "common things occur commonly" remains true for the immunocompromised host. Thus, perforation of a viscus, intestinal obstruction, acute cholecystitis, and diverticulitis may all be encountered in the immunocompromised. However, the astute clinician should have a high index of suspicion for specific problems associated with the patient's underlying disease, such as neutropenic enterocolitis in leukemic patients receiving chemotherapy, graft-versus-host disease in allogeneic bone marrow transplant recipients, perforation in patients with intestinal lymphomas receiving chemotherapy, cytomegalovirus (CMV) colitis in organ transplant recipients aggressively being treated for rejection, and intestinal obstruction secondary to Kaposi's sarcoma in an HIV-positive patient with cutaneous lesions. Often, prompt initiation of appropriate therapy, which includes antibiotic coverage for suspected pathogens, decreasing the immu-nosuppression in septic transplant recipients or, conversely, increasing the immunosuppression for graft-versus-host disease, may be lifesaving and provide a diagnosis either by exclusion or based on the response to therapy where a clear diagnosis cannot be established. Patients in whom immediate surgical intervention is not considered necessary must have frequent evaluations (several times a day) by the same physician to accurately assess the patient's response to initial medical management. Any worsening of symptoms or deterioration in clinical course should prompt surgical intervention. Thus, many problems that can initially be managed medically (eg, CMV colitis) may progress and later require surgical intervention (CMV-induced colonic perforation). Only by having the same person examine the patient frequently can this critical change be detected early and thereby maximize the chances of survival. Procrastination in the face of a complex clinical presentation and diagnostic uncertainty until there is full-blown abdominal sepsis is a grave error. It should be kept in mind that laparotomy may be used to advantage as part of the diagnostic evaluation and is remarkably well tolerated, even by these critically ill patients. On the other hand, a missed diagnosis of abdominal sepsis is likely to prove fatal. Thus, the surgeon should avoid a nihilistic approach, since many immunocompromised hosts have a good long-term prognosis if they are able to survive the acute event.

SPECIFIC DISEASES ASSOCIATED WITH THE IMMUNOCOMPROMISED STATE

Tuberculosis

The incidence of tuberculosis in the United States is rapidly increasing, mainly because of the AIDS pandemic and the large number of immigrants from countries where HIV is endemic. The immunocompromised state increases the risk for reactivation of latent tuberculous infection and for progressive disease from new infection. In HIV-infected patients, extrapulmonary tuberculosis is an AIDS-defining diagnosis that often precedes other opportunistic infections because of its increased virulence. Tuberculosis may also affect otherwise normal individuals, usually young women, who probably have a mild undetectable dysfunction of their cellular immune system.

Abdominal tuberculosis may involve the gastrointestinal tract as a result of swallowing infected sputum or contaminated milk. It may also involve the peritoneum by direct extension from another abdominal site or hematogenous spread from a pulmonary focus.

The commonest sites of intestinal involvement are the terminal ileum and ileocecal region, followed by the jejunum and colon. Approximately 75% of patients with gastrointestinal lesions will have evidence of current or past pulmonary tuberculosis. Purified protein derivative (PPD) tuberculin skin testing is positive in over half of mildly immunocompromised patients but will be negative in the anergic severely immunocompromised host. Thus, a positive skin test is helpful, but a negative test does not exclude the diagnosis. Distal small-intestinal obstruction caused by hypertrophic lesions or strictures is the most common presentation, followed by perforation. Ascites and subacute obstruction caused by adhesions also are common with peritoneal involvement. Symptoms are usually nonspecific and consist of colicky mid-abdominal and right lower quadrant pain reflecting intermittent partial intestinal obstruction. Fever, weight loss, and change in bowel habits are often present. Abdominal distention and a right lower quadrant mass are seen in advanced cases. Peripheral adenopathy is usually absent. Stool may be guaiac-positive, but frank bleeding is uncommon. Plain roentgenograms of the abdomen may show evidence of distal small-intestinal obstruction, calcified mesenteric lymph nodes, or calcification in the liver or spleen. Barium contrast studies of the upper or lower intestinal tract may reveal stenosis or ulceration involving the terminal ileum or elsewhere, which must be differentiated from carcinoma or regional enteritis.

In tuberculous peritonitis, the entire peritoneal surface is usually covered with 1- to 2-mm tubercles. It also presents insidiously, with mild abdominal pain and ascites being the most frequent findings. Fever and weight loss are also often present. Abdominal tenderness is mild to moderate, and tuberculous peritonitis rarely causes boardlike rigidity or rebound tenderness, as seen with bacterial peritonitis. Examination of peritoneal fluid reveals a protein- (greater than 2.5 g/100 mL) and lymphocyte- (greater than 50% of total white blood cells) rich ascites. Stains for acid-fast bacilli and cultures are often negative. Other opportunistic pathogens causing spontaneous peritonitis include *Mycobacterium avium-intracellulare* (MAI), *Cryptococcus neoformans*, and *Strongyloides*. Differentiation from peritoneal carcinomatosis may require cytologic examination of ascitic fluid or histologic examination of laparoscopic biopsy specimens.

MAI is a ubiquitous organism often found in the water supply, which has a low virulence and rarely causes disease in immunocompetent patients. In AIDS patients, disseminated MAI is a "late" opportunistic infection, since it typically presents in advanced cases with CD4$^+$ cell counts well below 200/mm^3. The clinical features of disseminated MAI infection are dominated by systemic symptoms of fever, weight loss, and diarrhea; bone lesions may cause localized pain. Physical findings are those of generalized involvement of the reticuloendothelial system with lymphadenopathy and hepatosplenomegaly. Gastrointestinal symptoms are uncommon except for chronic diarrhea.

Neutropenic Enterocolitis

Neutropenic enterocolitis, also known as typhlitis or ileocecal syndrome, is a recognized complication of chemotherapy for leukemia and other hematologic malignant diseases. It has also been reported in patients with aplastic anemia and cyclic neutropenia. Neutropenia appears to be the sine qua non of this syndrome. Pathologic findings are usually limited to the ileocecal region and consist of mucosal ulcerations and patchy areas of necrosis with bacterial or fungal invasion of the intestinal wall. The early clinical presentation consists of high fevers, nausea, vomiting, abdominal distention, and bloody diarrhea. Eventually abdominal pain localizes to the right lower quadrant and signs of peritoneal irritation are evident. Plain abdominal roentgenograms show decreased gas in the right lower quadrant and a dilated, fluid-filled intestine. Blood cultures are often positive for enteric and fungal pathogens. Although patients with early signs may be managed conservatively with intestinal decompression, intravenous antibiotics, hydration, and adjustments in their chemotherapy to allow reversal of the neutropenia, evidence of peritoneal irritation requires prompt exploration and resection of the involved segment.

Since many of these patients are young and have recently been on antibiotics, differentiation from acute appendicitis and pseudomembranous colitis is essential. Thus, right lower quadrant pain in a leukemic child who is not neutropenic suggests acute appendicitis, and operation should not be delayed. Also, all patients in whom the diagnosis of neutropenic enterocolitis is entertained require a sigmoidoscopy and stool samples for *Clostridium difficile* antigen and culture to exclude pseudomembranous colitis.

Graft-versus-Host Disease

Graft-versus-host disease (GVHD) occurs when allogeneic mature T cells are transplanted into an immunocompromised recipient who is incapable of destroying them (host-versus-graft reaction or rejection). The transplanted cells then recognize the host as foreign and initiate a graft-versus-host reaction. This sequence is seen in 10% to 80% of allogeneic bone marrow transplant recipients, depending on the degree of histoincompatibility, the number of T cells transplanted with the graft, the patient's age, and the prophylactic regimen. Although rarely seen, it may also occur in solid-organ transplant recipients, especially with liver and small-intestine transplantation, because of the large number of lymphoid cells contained within these allografts. The principal target organs are the immune system, skin, liver, and intestine. The importance of identifying GVHD as the cause of abdominal pain is that surgical intervention is not required unless a complication, such as perforation, has occurred.

Acute GVHD usually occurs within the first 2 months after transplantation. The skin is initially involved, presenting as a pruritic maculopapular rash over the palms, soles, and ears, progressing to total body erythroderma. Gastrointestinal and liver symptoms present later and rarely precede the skin lesions. Patients develop anorexia, vomiting, abdominal pain and distention with plain roentgenograms showing a paralytic ileus. The liver is usually not tender, but liver function tests reveal hyperbilirubinemia with elevation of alkaline phosphatase and amino transferase values. The host's immune system is also attacked by the foreign T cells, producing a state of profound immunodeficiency, which is accentuated by the immunosuppressive agents used to treat the GVHD. The patient then becomes susceptible to opportunistic infection, which may further complicate the clinical situation.

Chronic GVHD usually presents after the first 2 months following allogeneic bone marrow transplantation and may be a continuum of acute GVHD or present de novo. Skin changes, cholestatic liver disease, and immune deficiency are prominent; intestinal involvement is infrequent except for dysphagia secondary to a dry mouth (sicca syndrome) and severe mucositis involving the esophagus.

Finally, syngeneic GVHD has been described in recipients of autologous bone marrow transplants. This is a form of autoimmune disease that is self-limited and predominantly affects the skin. Thus, intestinal symptoms in these patients must not be attributed to GVHD, and a search must be made for complications of the underlying disease, the chemotherapy, or opportunistic infections.

Cytomegalovirus

CMV is a common pathogen in severely immunocompromised patients. Over 70% of the adult population has been infected with the virus, but disease usually occurs only in immunocompromised hosts. It can present as reactivation of a latent infection, superinfection with a new viral strain, or as a primary infection, which typically leads to a more severe form of the disease as seen in CMV-negative recipients of CMV-positive organ transplants. It is the most common opportunistic infection in bone marrow and solid-organ transplant recipients and causes clinically significant infection in over 50% of AIDS patients. It is important to differentiate CMV infection from CMV disease. CMV infection is very common and is asymptomatic. It is diagnosed by a fourfold increase in serum anti-CMV antibody titer or viral shedding. CMV disease implies tissue invasion and disease caused by the virus. Diagnosis requires demonstration of viral inclusions in biopsy specimens or positive cultures from blood, bronchoalveolar lavage fluid, or tissue biopsies.

Mild clinical manifestations of CMV disease consist of fever, malaise, and myalgias; leukopenia is often present. More severe disease can affect any organ system and present as retinitis, pneumonitis, hepatitis, acalculous cholecystitis, pancreatitis, or gastroenteritis—any of which can progress to multiple organ failure, sepsis, and death. CMV infects the endothelial cells of the intestinal mucosal capillaries, causing diffuse ischemic mucosal ulcerations, most often involving the terminal ileum and colon. Patients may present with diarrhea, evidence of lower gastrointestinal hemorrhage, or perforation. Evaluation must include an upper or lower gastrointestinal endoscopy with adequate mucosal biopsies. On endoscopy, numerous, well-circumscribed ulcerations with an overlying fibrinous exudate are visualized and may mimic pseudomembranous colitis. Biopsy reveals characteristic CMV inclusions in the endothelial cells. CMV disease usually does not require surgical intervention. Supportive care, administration of antiviral agents (eg, gancyclovir) and, for severe cases, reduction of the immunosuppressive medications are usually successful. Patients with massive lower gastrointestinal bleeding or evidence of perforation require prompt surgical intervention.

Kaposi's Sarcoma

Kaposi's sarcoma (KS) is a multifocal malignant disease that probably originates from vascular endothelial cells. Although originally described in elderly men of Jewish or Mediterranean descent and as an endemic disease in certain parts of Africa, the current epidemic is due to the increasing AIDS population. It has also been reported in renal transplant recipients and patients on steroids for autoimmune diseases. Over 30% of AIDS patients develop KS, and renal transplant recipients have a 400% to 500% greater incidence of KS than noted in the general population.

Cutaneous lesions range from minimally erythematous macules to the more obvious violaceous pigmented nodules and plaques. Typically, lesions involve the nose, periorbital skin, external ear, genitalia, and feet, but any cutaneous site may be involved. Intestinal involvement occurs in approximately 50% of AIDS patients with cutaneous lesions; in a few patients, intestinal lesions will precede the skin lesions. Any part of the intestinal tract from the oral cavity to the rectum may be involved; the spleen, liver, pancreas, and lymph nodes are also often involved. Intestinal lesions have a characteristic endoscopic appearance and present as violaceous macules or umbilicated nodules. Endoscopic biopsies of luminal lesions are unreliable because of their predominantly submucosal location; thus multiple biopsies from various sites are necessary. Bleeding from biopsy sites is rare.

Kaposi's sarcoma of the gastrointestinal tract is usually an incidental finding that infrequently causes symptoms. However, cases of massive intestinal bleeding, diarrhea, intestinal obstruction, and perforation have been reported. Of more significance clinically, KS of the intestinal tract is a sign of severe immunocompromise in patients often presenting with other opportunistic infections that must be diagnosed and treated adequately. This is especially true of patients receiving systemic chemotherapy for the treatment of disseminated KS. Also, α-interferon, often used in the treatment of KS, causes a "flulike" syndrome characterized by fevers, myalgias, confusion, nausea, diarrhea, elevated liver enzyme levels, and cytopenias, which must also be differentiated from opportunistic infections.

Lymphomas

The incidence of lymphoma is greatly increased in the immunocompromised host. The incidence increases with the degree of immunocompromise, being 1% for renal, 2% for heart, 3% for liver, and 4.6% for heart-lung transplant recipients; an actuarial risk as high as 46% is predicted for advanced AIDS victims. Contrary to the incidence in the general population, these are usually extranodal, high-grade, non-Hodgkin's B cell lymphomas, involving the central nervous system, gastrointestinal tract, bone marrow, and liver in decreasing order of frequency. The Epstein-Barr virus (EBV) appears to be the etiologic agent, initiating a polyclonal B-cell proliferation in a host with a defective cellular immune system incapable of containing the proliferative response, with progression to monoclonality.

In transplant recipients, lymphomas may develop as early as a few months posttransplant especially in patients receiving intensive induction-rejection regimens, which include antilymphocyte preparations (eg, OKT3).

In less intensely immunosuppressed allograft recipients, lymphomas usually present over 1 year after the transplant.

Although any segment or all of the gastrointestinal tract may be involved, the distal ileum is the most common site. Initial presentation may be as free perforation, gastrointestinal bleeding, obstruction, or a palpable mass. Since lymphomas are very sensitive to radiotherapy and chemotherapy, perforation or bleeding may also occur during treatment. Systemic symptoms of lymphoma, ie, unexplained fever, night sweats, or weight loss are often present and require a careful evaluation to exclude other intercurrent opportunistic infections that are especially common during the administration of intensive chemotherapeutic regimens.

Evaluation must include histologic confirmation of any lesions, since mycobacterial and fungal infections may also present as hepatic lesions, abdominal masses, or luminal defects; endoscopic biopsies or CT-guided needle biopsies are often diagnostic. Once the diagnosis is made, gallium scanning, head and abdominal CT, bone marrow aspiration, and lumbar puncture will help determine the extent of the disease.

SPECIFIC PROBLEMS IN DIFFERENT ORGANS

Esophagus

Immunocompromised patients are susceptible to opportunistic infections of the esophagus. *Candida albicans* is the most common organism isolated, but CMV, herpes simplex virus (HSV), HIV, *Torulopsis glabrata*, *Mycobacterium tuberculosis*, and *Cryptosporidium* have also been identified in esophageal lesions. Other possible causes of esophageal symptoms include zidovudine-induced ulcers or obstructive symptoms from lymphomas or Kaposi's sarcoma. Chronic GVHD may produce dysphagia caused by a dry mouth and severe mucositis. Since many of these agents produce similar superficial lesions and specific therapy is available for many of them, a definitive tissue diagnosis is imperative.

Complaints of dysphagia, odynophagia, or retrosternal pain warrant a careful evaluation. Severe cases may present as upper gastrointestinal hemorrhage or perforation with mediastinitis. Examination of the oropharynx may demonstrate the typical multifocal, curdlike plaques of candidiasis. These are usually easily removed by scraping with a tongue depressor; potassium hydroxide preparation reveals multiple blastospores and pseudohyphae. Once the diagnosis of oral candidiasis is confirmed, esophageal symptoms can be attributed to esophageal involvement and appropriate therapy initiated without further evaluation. Patients who fail to respond to initial therapy or are without evidence of oral candidiasis warrant an endoscopy, with biopsy of any esophageal lesions. Barium contrast studies are usually not helpful, since they may miss superficial erosions and cannot differentiate among the various etiologic agents.

Stomach

Gastroduodenal lesions are common in the immunocompromised patient and are usually manifested by hemorrhage, perforation, or obstruction. The adverse effects of gastric acid and pepsin on the gastric mucosa may be exacerbated by the use of steroids, which decrease the mucosal barrier; antimetabolites (azathioprine, methotrexate etc), which delay mucosal healing; and the presence of clotting abnormalities (uremia, thrombocytopenia), all of which predispose to hemorrhage and perforation. The widespread use of antacid prophylaxis has greatly reduced the complications of peptic ulcer disease in transplant recipients and other critically ill patients. Currently, opportunistic infections and malignant neoplasia are the most common causes of significant gastroduodenal lesions in the severely immunocompromised patient.

Hemorrhage, the most common significant symptom, is associated with high mortality. CMV and lymphomas are usually the underlying problems, but *Candida* ulcers, Kaposi's sarcoma, leukemic infiltrates, and other opportunistic infections must also be considered. Patients receiving chemotherapy are especially susceptible to hemorrhage or perforation of their malignant lesions. Unlike the general population, in which peptic ulcer disease is the presumed cause of upper gastrointestinal bleeding, immunocompromised patients require early endoscopy and biopsy for definitive diagnosis and institution of appropriate therapy.

Perforation, as evidenced by epigastric or diffuse abdominal pain, board-like abdomen and evidence of free air under the diaphragm requires prompt surgical intervention. At times patients may present with few symptoms and evidence of pneumoperitoneum on upright chest or abdominal roentgenograms as the only significant finding. Gastric outlet obstruction with epigastric fullness and abilious vomitus is an indication for endoscopy and biopsy, since malignant lesions are often the underlying problem.

Small Intestine

The small intestine is often involved by opportunistic infections and malignant disease in immunocompromised hosts. The site of involvement increases in frequency from the ligament of Treitz to the terminal ileum. Clinically, patients may present with diarrhea, bleeding, perforation, or obstruction, often but not necessarily associated with fever, leukocytosis, and abdominal pain. Diarrhea is especially common in AIDS patients and warrants a prompt and thorough evaluation so that specific therapy can be administered before complications occur. In most instances, patients with abdominal pain and diarrhea do not require operative therapy. On the other hand, if an underlying infectious cause is not identified and treated promptly, complications requiring surgical intervention, such as massive lower intestinal bleeding or perforation, may ensue.

Cryptosporidium, MAI, and *Isospora belli* are the most common stool isolates involving the jejunoileum in AIDS patients with diarrhea; CMV is also a common pathogen in AIDS and other severely immunosuppressed patients. Other pathogens affecting the colon, eg, *C difficile* toxin and *Entamoeba histolytica,* must also be considered. Medications such as DDI and OKT3 may also produce diarrhea and must be considered in the differential diagnosis. Finally, the HIV virus itself may infect the gastrointestinal tract, producing a chronic diarrhea with malabsorption (AIDS enteropathy).

Evaluation of immunocompromised patients with diarrhea includes examination of stool for ova and parasites, stool cultures for common pathogens (*Shigella, Salmonella, Campylobacter,* etc.), stool *C difficile* culture and toxin assay, and sigmoidoscopy or colonoscopy with appropriate biopsies. In certain cases, upper gastrointestinal endoscopy and biopsy may identify CMV or MAI; also duodenal aspirates may identify *Giardia lamblia* trophozoites. Although stool cultures are often positive for *Candida,* these are usually not significant unless tissue invasion is shown on mucosal biopsy specimens.

As described with gastric lesions, small-intestinal obstruction, bleeding, or perforation is often due to opportunistic malignant diseases (lymphomas and Kaposi's sarcoma) or opportunistic infections (mycobacteria, CMV, etc), which must be considered in the differential diagnosis. Because of the diffuse intestinal involvement with many of these diseases, upper or lower intestinal endoscopy with appropriate mucosal biopsies may be diagnostic. Plain abdominal roentgenograms and contrast studies may help identify an obstruction or perforation but will not differentiate the possible etiologies. At the time of laparotomy, appropriate culture and pathologic examination of any enlarged lymph nodes and resected intestine will help identify the underlying problem and determine further management.

Colon

As with the rest of the gastrointestinal tract, the colon is also often involved with opportunistic infections and malignant tumors in the immunocompromised host and may present as bleeding, perforation, or obstruction. Furthermore, specific entities such as acute appendicitis, diverticulitis, fecal impaction, and colonic pseudo-obstruction (Ogilvie's syndrome) must also be considered.

Colonic perforation usually occurs in the sigmoid and is secondary to diverticulitis, especially in the renal transplant population, where the prevalence of diverticulosis is high. Other common etiologies include ischemic colitis, fecal impaction, opportunistic infections (CMV, *Candida*), pseudomembranous colitis, and malignant disease. Patients present with abdominal pain, fever, and signs of peritoneal irritation on physical examination; leukocytosis is variably present. Because of the patient's inability to localize the inflammatory process, pneumoperitoneum is seen on plain chest or abdominal roentgenograms in over 90% of cases.

Lower gastrointestinal bleeding in transplant recipients is often due to opportunistic infections (CMV, *Candida*) producing ulcerations of the cecum or other segments of the gastrointestinal tract. This usually occurs in the first few months after transplantation, when the patient is overimmunosuppressed during treatment of a rejection episode. Also, common causes of lower gastrointestinal bleeding such as diverticulosis and malignant lesions must also be considered. The presence of bloody diarrhea suggests other etiologies, such as ischemic colitis, pseudomembranous colitis, exacerbation of inflammatory bowel disease symptoms, amebiasis, or shigellosis. Stool samples for microscopic examination, culture, and *C difficile* toxin assay, plus lower intestinal endoscopy with appropriate biopsies are essential for an adequate diagnosis.

Colonic obstruction occurs infrequently in the immunocompromised patient. Common causes such as sigmoid adenocarcinoma, diverticulitis, or volvulus must be considered. Other possible etiologies often found in immunocompromised patients include fecal impaction and Kaposi's sarcoma. Patients usually present with obstipation and nontender abdominal distention. Abdominal roentgenograms reveal colonic distention extending from the cecum distally to the site of obstruction. If the ileocecal valve is incompetent, the small intestine will also be distended. A history of chronic constipation, recent abdominal surgery, use of constipating analgesics, uremia, or diabetes is often present in cases of fecal impaction, which will often involve the right colon. In AIDS patients, the presence of Kaposi's sarcoma elsewhere should raise suspicion of colonic involvement.

Mechanical colonic obstruction, which requires surgical intervention, must be differentiated from pseudo-obstruction of the colon (Ogilvie's syndrome). Pseudo-obstruction of the colon is often seen in hospitalized patients with other severe medical illnesses. These patients present with symptoms of colonic obstruction without having a mechanical obstruction. The setting is often that of a severely ill patient with electrolyte abnormalities, possibly receiving constipating analgesics, who develops painless abdominal distention. The presence of watery diarrhea may suggest the absence of a mechanical obstruction. A full colonoscopy can be both diagnostic and therapeutic. The presence of bloody diarrhea suggests other diagnoses, such as toxic megacolon.

Acute appendicitis is uncommon in the immunocompromised patient, probably because of atrophy of the submucosal lymphoid follicles thought to be responsible for the obstruction and subsequent infection of the appendix. Despite this generalization, acute appendicitis must be considered in the differential diagnosis of any patient, especially a child, with right lower quadrant pain.

Also, in AIDS patients, other diseases such as CMV infection, Kaposi's sarcoma, or lymphomas may obstruct the appendix. Patients often present with progressive right lower quadrant pain and diarrhea; fever and leukocytosis are not always present. Because of the numerous intestinal problems seen in immunocompromised patients, an abdominal ultrasonogram may aid in the diagnosis and avoid undue delays in treatment. In renal transplant recipients, in whom the allograft is also in the right lower quadrant, severe acute rejection may present with a similar picture. A rapidly rising serum creatinine will suggest this latter diagnosis.

Pancreas

Acute pancreatitis is uncommon in immunocompromised hosts but carries a high mortality. As well as the abuse of alcohol and gallstones, other processes are often responsible for the acute episode.

In renal transplant recipients, hypercalcemia, hyperlipidemia, high-dose steroids, azathioprine, and CMV infection are other possible etiologies. In AIDS patients, the use of DDI and intravenous pentamidine have been implicated in the rising incidence of pancreatitis in this patient population. Opportunistic infections with CMV, *Cryptococcus*, and *Toxoplasma gondii* have also been reported to cause pancreatitis in AIDS patients.

As in the general population, patients usually present with upper abdominal pain, nausea, and vomiting; diffuse abdominal pain with ileus and cardiovascular collapse is seen in severe cases. A CT scan with infusion helps confirm the diagnosis when in doubt and determine the extent of necrosis in severe cases. Elevated levels of serum amylase and lipase are suggestive, but other causes of hyperamylasemia such as bowel perforation must also be considered. It must be remembered that amylase is excreted in the urine so that dialysis patients often have mild hyperamylasemia (less than 300 U/L). Also, asymptomatic hyperamylasemia has been observed after renal transplantation. It is probably related to high-dose steroids and is self-limited.

Although the pancreas is often involved by disseminated opportunistic neoplasms, the lesions are usually asymptomatic and only identified at autopsy.

Biliary Tract Disease

As in the general population, fever, right upper quadrant pain, leukocytosis, and a cholestatic biochemical profile are the presenting symptoms of biliary tract disease in immunocompromised patients. Besides cholecystitis caused by gallstones, acalculous cholecystitis is commonly seen in immunocompromised patients. Acalculous cholecystitis is usually seen in older (over 50 years) men with critical illnesses, trauma, or major unrelated operations often associated with prolonged fasting and parenteral nutrition. In severely immunocompromised patients and especially in young AIDS patients, opportunistic infections of the gallbladder and biliary tree can give rise to acalculous cholecystitis and cholangitis. CMV, *Cryptosporidium*, and *Microsporida* have often been identified in bile cultures or biopsy specimens. Also, external compression of the biliary tree by enlarged lymph nodes (MAI, lymphoma, etc) or direct invasion by neoplasms (Kaposi's sarcoma) may present as cholecystitis or cholangitis. Patients often present with unexplained fever and later develop the other localizing signs and symptoms. The presence of chronic diarrhea suggests acalculous cholecystitis by opportunistic organisms. Ultrasonographic examination of the right upper quadrant may point to the correct diagnosis. For acalculous cholecystitis, one of the following ultrasonographic signs is present in over 90% of cases: (1) thickened gallbladder wall (greater than 3 mm); (2) an enlarged, tender gallbladder, and (3) a pericholecystic fluid collection suggestive of a localized perforation. The presence of ascites or chronic cholecystitis limits the usefulness of these three criteria. Nonvisualization of the gallbladder on radionuclide scans (HIDA, DISIDA, etc) is less helpful because of the high incidence of false-positive results in fasting patients.

Patients with a clinical picture suggestive of biliary tract disease should have an abdominal ultrasonogram. The presence of gallstones or any of the three ultrasonographic signs of acalculous cholecystitis are indications for prompt cholecystectomy owing to the rapid progression to gallbladder necrosis and perforation. If none of the above are present and there is evidence of biliary tree dilatation, endoscopic retrograde cholangio-pancreatography (ERCP) will allow for an anatomic diagnosis, sampling bile for cultures and tissue for biopsies of the ampulla. Biopsy may reveal CMV, *Cryptosporidium*, other pathogens, or neoplasia. The so called AIDS cholangiopathy refers to a spectrum of biliary tract disorders, including papillary stenosis, sclerosing cholangitis, and long extrahepatic bile duct strictures. All of these can be identified with ERCP and are secondary to opportunistic infections and chronic inflammation. Patients with a normal ultrasonogram warrant a liver biopsy.

Liver and Spleen

Liver disease is often manifested by fever, hepatosplenomegaly, right upper quadrant pain, and abnormal liver chemistries. In transplant recipients and intravenous drug abusers, hepatitis B and C are the most common viral pathogens. Also, in all severely immunocompromised patients, CMV is a common cause of hepatitis. Other opportunistic pathogens that may involve the liver include MAI, *Cryptococcus neoformans*, *Histoplasma capsulatum*, *Microsporida*, *Toxoplasma gondii*, and *Listeria monocytogenes*. Finally, *Candida* is the most common cause of liver abscesses in immunosuppressed patients; *Aspergillus* and amebas are less common.

Patients with right upper quadrant pain and abnormal liver chemistries are evaluated as described for biliary tract disease. A normal ultrasonogram is an indication for a liver biopsy; if an abscess is suspected, CT-guided aspiration can be both diagnostic and therapeutic.

Hepatic venoocclusive disease can occur in the first few weeks after bone marrow transplantation and presents as right upper quadrant pain, hepatomegaly, ascites, and jaundice. It can be differentiated from acute GVHD involving the liver, since weight gain and right upper quadrant pain are rare occurrences with GVHD. Liver involvement by Kaposi's sarcoma or lymphoma, although common, is usually asymptomatic.

Splenomegaly secondary to neoplastic involvement (leukemia, lymphoma, Kaposi's sarcoma) or abscesses (*Candida*, MAI, *M tuberculosis*) often presents as left upper quadrant pain or signs of sepsis. Splenic rupture is also possible. A CT scan will help to identify the problem. Abscesses can be aspirated for an accurate diagnosis.

CONCLUSIONS

The immunocompromised patient is susceptible to numerous opportunistic infections and neoplasms, often occurring simultaneously, which must be considered in the differential diagnosis of abdominal pain. A high index of suspicion and an aggressive evaluation are essential for an accurate diagnosis so that unnecessary surgical interventions and fatal delays when surgery is indicated can be avoided.

SUGGESTED READING

Alt B, Glass NR, Sollinger H. Neutropenic enterocolitis in adults: review of literature and assessment of surgical intervention. *Am J Surg.* 1985; 149:405.

Bastani B, Shariatzadeh MR, Dehdashti F. Tuberculous peritonitis—report of 30 cases and review of the literature. *Q. J Med.* 1985; 221:549.

Dunn DL. Problems related to immunosuppression: infection and malignancy occurring after solid organ transplantation. *Crit Care Clin* 1990; 6:955.

Glen J, Funkhouser WK, Schneider PS. Acute illnesses necessitating urgent abdominal surgery in neutropenic cancer patients: description of 14 cases and review of the literature. *Surgery.* 1989; 105:778.

Nylander WA. The acute abdomen in the immunocompromised host. *Surg Clin North Am.* 1988; 68:457.

Pollak R, Jonasson O. Surgery in the immunocompromised patient. *Probl Gen Surg.* 1984; 1:390.

Potter DA, Danforth DN, Macher AM, et al. Evaluation of abdominal pain in the AIDS patient. *Ann Surg.* 1984; 199:332.

Schaller RT, Schaller JF. The acute abdomen in the immunologically compromised child. *J Pediatr Surg* 1983; 18:937.

Sievert W, Merrell RC. Gastrointestinal emergencies in the acquired immunodeficiency syndrome. *Gastroenteral Clin North Am.* 1988; 17:409.

Tanowitz HB, Simon D, Wittner M. Medical management of AIDS patients: gastrointestinal manifestations. *Med Clin North Am.* 1992; 76:45.

CHAPTER 16

■

Nonsurgical Causes of Abdominal Pain

Joseph M. Vitello, MD

Acute abdominal pain is not always caused by a process resulting in peritonitis or intra-abdominal hemorrhage. In fact, the problem may be remote from the abdomen. There exist a variety of extra-abdominal disorders that, while presenting with abdominal pain, have little or no surgical significance. The astute physician must be able to recognize those processes that manifest themselves partly or entirely as abdominal pain, yet do not require the surgeon's knife. In some instances, operation is even meddlesome and may worsen the condition. In other situations, however, the diagnosis is so confusing and difficult that viewing the abdominal contents is the definitive diagnostic test. In this case, even though the decision to operate may have been erroneous, no apology is necessary. Table 14 offers a list of the more commonly encountered problems in this category, and the majority are discussed below.

RESPIRATORY SYSTEM

Infections of the upper respiratory tract, especially in children, are often associated with abdominal pain and vomiting. Usually there is no associated muscular rigidity, although the children are crying and tense and give the illusion of an abdominal crisis.

Hospitalization with repeated abdominal examination by the same observer will invariably solve the problem and reveal no localizing abdominal findings. An important point is that the same examiner should reevaluate the patient. Once rapport has been developed between physician and patient, subsequent serial examinations are easily understood as essential to quality care and are not perceived as bothersome. This point has greater importance

TABLE 14. NONSURGICAL CAUSES OF ABDOMINAL PAIN

System	Disease or Disorder
Pulmonary	Pneumonia
	Pleurisy
	Influenza
	Pulmonary embolus or infarction
	Spontaneous pneumothorax
Cardiovascular	Myocardial ischemia or infarction
	Congestive heart failure
	Pericarditis
	Thoracic aortic dissection*
	Mesenteric vascular insufficiency*
	Ischemic colitis*
	Periarteritis nodosa
	Systemic lupus erythematosus
	Schönlein-Henoch purpura*
Genitourinary	Renal or ureteral colic
	Pyelonephritis
	Cystitis
	Testicular torsion
	Epididymitis
	Acute urinary retention
Gastrointestinal	Gastritis
	Food poisoning
	Bacterial or viral gastroenteritis
	Lactose intolerance
	Mesenteric adenitis
	Inflammatory bowel diseases*
	Pseudomembranous enterocolitis*
	Allergic abdominal pain
	Constipation
	Irritable bowel syndrome
	Cystic fibrosis
	Organomegaly
	Adhesions(?)*
Hematopoietic	Lymphoma*
	Leukemia
	Splenic rupture*
	Sickle-cell crises
	Hemolytic-uremic syndrome
	Coagulation disorders (acquired and hereditary)
Neuromuscular and skeletal	Herpes zoster (shingles)
	Herniated nucleus pulposus
	Spinal cord neoplasm or space-occupying lesion
	Nerve entrapment syndrome
	Periostitis pubis
	Abdominal wall hernias*
	Spider bites
	Rectus sheath hematoma

TABLE 14. (*Continued*)

System	Disease or Disorder
Metabolic and endocrine	Diabetic ketoacidosis
	Lead poisoning
	Adrenal insufficiency
	Porphyria
	Primary hyperparathyroidism
	Familial Mediterranean fever
	Thyroid storm (thyrotoxicosis)
	Electrolyte depletion
	Hereditary angioneurotic edema
	Hyperlipoproteinemia types I, V
	Drug addiction: Withdrawal
All systems: infectious diseases	Malaria
	Tuberculosis*
	Typhoid
	Syphilis
	Primary peritonitis
	Hepatitis
	Trichinosis
	Amebiasis*
	Ascariasis
	Rheumatic fever
	Whipples's disease
	Rocky Mountain spotted fever
	Fitz-Hugh-Curtis syndrome (gonococcal perihepatitis)*

*Diseases that may have an abdominal surgical component.

in a teaching hospital, where many medical students, various levels of residents, and attending physicians are intricately involved in patient care. In all the following circumstances, while abdominal pain may be part of the initial presentation, a thorough evaluation of the pulmonary system by physical examination and roentgenography will delineate these entities from true abdominal pathologic processes.

Pneumonia

Pneumonia may cause abdominal pain, tenderness, and even muscular rigidity. As a rule, this disease is not difficult to diagnose, as signs of pulmonary pathology such as shortness of breath, productive sputum, or rales can usually be demonstrated, if the examiner makes the effort. When there are no clear-cut findings of pulmonic disease, a chest roentgenogram usually clarifies the situation. It is essential to obtain an upright posterior-anterior and lateral chest radiograph before planned operation on any patient being evaluated with abdominal pain. Right lower lobe pneumonia can present with abdominal pain similar to acute cholecystitis or appendicitis. With pneumonia, the fever and leukocytosis tend to be more elevated than with appendicitis or cholecystitis. In the elderly, pneumonia may present with abdominal pain as the chief complaint. Plain roentgenograms of the abdomen may demonstrate a reflex ileus.

Pleurisy

Pleurisy, by irritating the diaphragm, may produce abdominal pain. The discomfort, which is occasionally severe, is worsened by a deep inspiration. A pleural friction rub may be detected on auscultation of the lungs. The chest roentgenogram is normal during the acute attack. The pleura is thickened if the process is chronic, as may occur in tuberculosis or asbestosis.

Pulmonary Embolism

Rarely, a pulmonary embolus may present with apparent abdominal pain, especially if a pulmonary infarct has occurred. However, given the circumstances of a patient on bed rest with risk factors such as obesity, malignant disease, or recent surgery and the atypical nature of the pain, a true abdominal source for the pain should be easy to exclude. Guarding and peritoneal signs are absent and pulmonary symptoms usually dominate the situation. Rales, wheezing, or a rub may be auscultated in a patient who is dyspneic and hypoxic.

Spontaneous Pneumothorax

Spontaneous pneumothorax can begin with severe, poorly localized pain similar to a perforated ulcer. With pneumothorax, however, the pain diminishes after the initial event. Dyspnea and chest discomfort then predominate. Auscultation and percussion of the involved hemithorax quickly clarifies any confusion and places the diagnosis on the proper side of the diaphragm. A chest roentgenogram confirms the diagnosis.

Influenza

Influenza can begin with abdominal pain, nausea, vomiting, and a fever. Initially, pronounced guarding may be noted on palpation of the abdomen, which can be misinterpreted as peritonitis. Malaise is a common accompaniment. Coryza and respiratory symptoms soon predominate. Serial examination will ultimately fail to show localizing abdominal tenderness.

CARDIOVASCULAR AND RELATED DISORDERS

Acute Myocardial Infarction

Angina pectoris or acute myocardial infarction (MI) usually produces pain posterior to the sternum, with radiation to the left arm and shoulder. However, the pain of an acute MI, on occasion, is felt primarily or entirely in the epigastrium. Often the patient believes the symptoms are due to dietary indiscretion and will be relieved with antacids or vomiting. The pain is often preceded by exertion and associated with anxiety. The patient may want to sit up, in contrast to the patient with peritonitis who wishes to lie still and flat. The discomfort is severe enough so that when not relieved over the course of several hours, medical attention is sought. The sudden, hyperacute onset of the pain makes a perforating ulcer, pancreatitis, cholecystitis, or a high, strangulated small-intestinal obstruction also suspect. However, physical findings in the abdomen rarely reveal any tenderness, rigidity, or rebound. If the cardiac evaluation is negative, an ultrasonogram of the gallbladder should be obtained in search of cholelithiasis, since this is commonly uncovered during the evaluation of "chest pain." If the electrocardiogram (ECG) or cardiac enzymes are abnormal, the diagnosis is secure, but cardiac angiography or stress testing may be necessary to exclude a cardiac source of pain.

Congestive Heart Failure
In acute congestive heart failure, venous stasis and passive congestion occur within the liver and other viscera. This can lead to right upper quadrant (RUQ) pain and the illusion of cholecystitis, hepatitis, or pancreatitis. Anorexia, nausea, and vomiting may also be prominent. There is minimal radiation of the pain and no rigidity or rebound. Jugular venous distention, hepatojugular reflex, and an S_3 gallop should be sought. Patients may display other evidence of heart failure including tachycardia, shortness of breath, and rales in the lung fields. The sclera may be icteric. In addition, acute cardiac decompensation may result in gastric dilatation or paralytic ileus, which may present as abdominal distention and pain.

Pericarditis
Acute pericarditis can produce fever, epigastric pain, and nausea. The cardiac signs can mimic those of infarction, or if there is an effusion, evidence of congestive heart failure will be present. A rub may be auscultated. The ECG may show ST segment elevation across all the precordial leads. The differentiation of pericarditis from a primary intra-abdominal process is generally based on the discrepancy between subjective abdominal complaints and objective findings.

Thoracic Aortic Dissection
A thoracic aortic dissection causes severe, tearing pain of sudden onset arising in the upper chest and back and progressing downward toward the abdomen. The predominance of back and chest pain seldom leads to diagnostic confusion, but occasionally epigastric complaints may predominate. The patients are usually older, with a history of long-standing hypertension, but thoracic aortic dissection may occur in a younger population as a result of cystic medial necrosis of the aorta. The femoral pulses may be diminished or ab-

sent. A variety of neurologic findings, including paralysis, may be noted if blood supply to the spinal cord is compromised. The murmur of aortic insufficiency may be detected. A chest roentgenogram reveals a widened mediastinum.

Mesenteric Vascular Insufficiency

Mesenteric vascular insufficiency (abdominal angina) is characterized by mild to moderate postprandial cramps, diarrhea, and eventually weight loss as a result of the patient's fear of eating and the precipitation of pain. The problem is a chronic one, the complaints vague, and there is usually no confusion with an acute abdominal catastrophe. No abdominal guarding or rebound exists, although there may be mild epigastric tenderness. The degree of pain may seem out of proportion to the objective findings. A bruit may be auscultated. The patients tend to be older and have other evidence of atherosclerosis. These patients usually have several emergency department or physician's office visits without objective findings. Many have been evaluated extensively and labeled neurotic. Biplanar celiac angiography is necessary to confirm the diagnosis by revealing a narrowed superior mesenteric artery. While the ultimate treatment may be surgical, emergency operation without the appropriate diagnostic evaluation will be unrevealing.

A second type of mesenteric ischemia leading to abdominal pain is the "low-flow state." This tends to occur in the hospitalized, critically ill patient. Predisposing factors include hemodynamic instability with reduced cardiac output from sepsis, myocardial infarction, dialysis, or hypovolemia. Drugs causing mesenteric vasoconstriction include digitalis, catecholamines, and vasopressin.

Ischemic colitis is a form of limited mesenteric ischemia. It may present with striking abdominal pain, leukocytosis, and evidence of peritonitis. Treatment, however, may be entirely supportive without the need for operation (85%), although progression of the disease may mandate resection. The diagnosis is established by identification of the population at risk and physical examination aided by endoscopic examination of the colon. The involved segment may be anywhere from cecum to sigmoid but most commonly involves the region of the splenic flexure. The ischemia tends to be mucosal and not transmural; therefore angiography is not essential, but endoscopy is mandatory. Current treatment includes bowel rest, parenteral nutrition, and hydration and antibiotics.

Periarteritis Nodosa

Periarteritis nodosa may give rise to severe abdominal pain and fever. The arteritis associated with this collagen disorder may involve the mesenteric vessels. In some patients, the pain is due to occlusion of small arteries leading to ischemia or infarction of the intestine or rupture of arterioles, causing focal mesenteric hemorrhage. In other patients, no source of pain can be identified.

The pain is often centrally located but may occur anywhere in the abdomen. Findings vary from mild distention and tenderness to an acute abdomen with signs of peritonitis. If pancreatic vessels are involved, acute pancreatitis may be precipitated. The diagnosis is difficult but should be suspected based on myalgias, polyarthritis, and elevated sedimentation rate. Treatment for periarteritis nodosa commonly includes steroids, which can be implicated in perforating ulcers and mask findings of other acute surgical problems.

Systemic Lupus Erythematosus

Systemic lupus erythematosus can be complicated by abdominal pain for a variety of reasons. Sometimes pain occurs without an obvious cause, other times it may be due to intestinal ulceration or pancreatitis. The tenderness is usually generalized. Rebound pain may be present. Anorexia, nausea, and vomiting frequently accompany the pain. Athralgias and arthritis with an elevated sedimentation rate are noted. The disease has a predilection for younger women. The characteristic butterfly rash in the malar distribution may be noted and 75% will have renal involvement manifested as azotemia. The diagnosis is confirmed with a positive antinuclear antibody test and demonstration of lupus erythematosus cells in the buffy coat of white cells.

Schönlein-Henoch Purpura

Schönlein-Henoch purpura (SHP) is seen most commonly in young children, but it also occurs in adults. It is a syndrome of unknown etiology but probably is related to an autoimmune disorder involving an IgA immune complex and small-vessel vasculitis. It is accompanied by abdominal pain, skin petechiae that coalesce into a palpable purpura, and small hemorrhages into a variety of tissues, most notably the kidneys and joints. An antecedent upper respiratory tract infection is noted in many patients 2 to 3 weeks before overt symptoms. The disease is usually self-limiting and mortality is rare, with most deaths attributed to nephritis. Skin manifestations occur in 100% of the patients, although they may not be present initially. The rash is usually seen on the buttocks and lower extremities. Arthralgia is the second most common manifestation of the illness (85%) and is usually monoarticular and generally affects the ankles or knees. Orchitis with hemorrhage and edema occurs in 2% to 38% of males with SHP and can mimic torsion. Gastrointestinal symptoms are common and occur in up to 75% of patients; however, surgical complications are rare, occurring only 2% to 6% of the time. Nausea and vomiting are seen frequently. The abdominal pain may precede the purpura and mimic the findings of appendicitis, peptic ulcer disease, or Crohn's disease, in which case an unnecessary operation may ensue. The pain is severe and sudden in onset, colicky, and may be followed by bloody diarrhea. This symptom complex suggests intussusception, and this is the most common surgical complication of SHP. Perforations of the gastrointestinal tract have also been reported, involving the stomach or small intestine or as a complication of the intussusception. The abdominal pain frequently results from submucosal and subserosal hemorrhage and edema resulting from the vasculitis. Laboratory data may also reveal a thrombocytosis, which has been noted in 90% of patients afflicted. The key to the diagnosis is recognition of the petechial rash, since in its absence, the findings suggest a surgical problem. At laparotomy the small intestine may be edematous and look intensely reddened from submucosal hemorrhages.

GENITOURINARY SYSTEM

Diseases of the kidney and urinary tract can give rise to severe abdominal pain because of overlap of autonomic innervation between genitourinary structures and other abdominal viscera. They must be considered in the patient with abdominal complaints.

Renal and Ureteral Colic

Renal and ureteral colic is accompanied by profuse nausea and vomiting with intense colicky pain. The pain usually begins in the lumbar region and radiates to the inguinal area toward the pubis or ipsilateral genitalia. The intensity of the pain is quite severe. Patients are writhing and unable to get comfortable, no matter which position they assume. This is in contrast to peritonitis, in which patients prefer to lie motionless. There is usually difficulty in voiding. The physical examination may show mild to moderate abdominal tenderness without peritonitis. There is costovertebral tenderness if the stone is lodged high in the ureter or renal pelvis. An ileus may develop with abdominal distention. There may be a low-grade temperature, and pulse and blood pressure are elevated from agitation and pain. Gross or microscopic hematuria is commonly found, although it may be absent with complete obstruction of a ureter. An intravenous urogram confirms the diagnosis.

Pyelonephritis

Uncomplicated pyelonephritis may cause acute pain of a dull nature in the groin or flank. Pyelonephritis is commonly associated with a high spiking fever, chills, rigors, and urinary frequency. The pain may be perceived as intra-abdominal, or a reflex ileus may lead to abdominal distention. Urinalysis usually demonstrates protein, white cells, occasionally red cells and bacteria in the sediment. With a perinephric abscess the patient usually has bacteremia and is septic without an obvious source. Posterior peritoneal irritation from a developing renal carbuncle can mimic retrocecal appendicitis, diverticulitis, or cholecystitis, although in most patients the pain localizes to the involved flank. Irritation of the iliohypogastric or genitofemoral nerves may refer pain to the hip, lower abdomen, or groin.

Cystitis

Cystitis usually gives rise to urgency, intense dysuria, and an abnormal urinalysis. The urine may have a foul smell, be cloudy in appearance, and be nitrite-positive on a dipstick test. Patients may complain of lower abdominal pain, which tends to localize in a suprapubic location. The lack of striking abdominal findings and the abnormal urine are enough to secure the diagnosis.

Torsion of the Testes

Abdominal pain as the initial manifestation of a testicular torsion is reported in 25% to 50% of patients. In this situation the pain is confined to the lower abdomen or inguinal areas but may be localized in the upper abdomen. Nausea, vomiting, and anorexia are common, but fever is not. Testicular torsion is a surgical emergency. Failure to have the patient undress fully and to perform a genital examination may result in a child's being admitted only for observation of abdominal pain. Torsion of a testicular appendage may present similarly to torsion of a testis.

Epididymitis

Acute epididymitis usually presents with testicular pain, but occasionally there is abdominal or inguinal pain and fever. Elevation of the testicle will relieve the pain and helps to differentiate this from torsion.

Urinary Retention

Acute urinary retention can give rise to severe pain in the lower abdomen. The distended bladder can extend to the umbilicus and be readily palpable and exquisitely tender. Any infraumbilical midline mass should be treated by urinary catheterization and reevaluation.

GASTROINTESTINAL DISORDERS

Gastritis

Gastritis is caused by ingestion of alcohol, aspirin, or other nonsteroidal medications or by excessive ingestion of certain foods. The symptoms of burning epigastric or griping midabdominal pain and nausea are not often confused with those of an acute surgical abdomen. There is usually no muscular rigidity or rebound tenderness and bowel sounds tend to be normal. Serial abdominal examinations reveal no localizing signs.

Food Poisoning

Food poisoning results from consuming contaminated food. The most common agent is the exotoxin of *Staphylococcus*, which typically does not alter the foods' taste. Symptoms occur within 8 hours of ingestion and are predominated by profuse vomiting, retching, and explosive diarrhea. Pain is due to the episodic, spasmodic hyperperistalsis, which leads to intense, crampy, periumbilical pain. These waves of pain are reminiscent of an intestinal obstruction, but the frequent watery stool and the history usually provide the clue to the diagnosis. Rebound pain or rigidity do not occur, although mild to moderate diffuse tenderness may predominate. Symptoms usually resolve within 24 hours. Food poisoning usually affects more than one person, and this valuable epidemiologic information should be sought.

Bacterial Gastroenteritis

Bacterial gastroenteritis occurs most commonly with *Salmonella, Shigella, Yersinia,* or strains of *Esherichia coli.* Colicky, occasionally severe abdominal pain, usually periumbilical in location, occurs suddenly. Nausea, vomiting, and diarrhea are prominent. The diarrhea may be bloody. Temperature elevation may be striking and occurs early in the course of the disease. In some instances, the pain may be localized to the right lower quadrant (RLQ) suggesting appendicitis. *Yersinia* infections have been implicated in acute appendicitis and a peculiar polyarthritic syndrome occasionally accompanied by erythema nodosum. In general, the diarrhea predominates and the abdominal findings are mild, without rebound. The bowel sounds are distinctly hyperactive. The white blood cell count is usually elevated and leukocytes in the stool may aid in the diagnosis. Stool cultures are needed to confirm the pathogen.

Malabsorption of Lactose

The malabsorption of lactose may result in intermittent abdominal pain. Intolerance occurs because of lactase deficiency, which increases with age. Unabsorbed disaccharide causes net secretion of electrolytes and water into the lumen of the small intestine. Upon reaching the colon, the sugar undergoes bacterial fermentation, producing gas, bloating, crampy pain, and diarrhea. Elimination of lactose from the diet improves the symptoms.

Mesenteric Adenitis

Mesenteric adenitis is a disease of adolescents, probably infectious, which causes anorexia and abdominal pain resembling acute appendicitis. Pain is greatest in the RLQ. This localization is related to the ileocolic mesenteric lymph nodes (Peyer's patches), which are enlarged in this process. Mesenteric adenitis often follows an upper respiratory tract infection or a bout of otitis media. While the pain may be quite severe, there is rarely rebound tenderness. The fever tends to be higher than with uncomplicated appendicitis. The white blood cell count frequently shows an absolute lymphocytosis rather than a left shift. If RLQ tenderness persists, exploration is warranted and if mesenteric adenitis is found, incidental appendectomy is reasonable.

Regional Enteritis

Regional enteritis (Crohn's disease) may involve any portion of the gastrointestinal tract but occasionally will affect only the terminal ileum and mimic acute appendicitis. There may be a family history of the disease. Diarrhea, which may be grossly bloody, cramps, and diffuse pain dominate the clinical situation. On occasion this has been confused with amebic colitis. If a barium study is obtained, it may reveal a "string sign" or a narrowed segment of terminal ileum. Most instances, however, present with RLQ tenderness and appendicitis is suspected.

Ulcerative Colitis

Ulcerative colitis is clinically similar to regional enteritis except it is confined to the colon and rectum. Crampy abdominal pain and bloody diarrhea herald the onset or exacerbation in known cases. The abdominal examination usually reveals diffuse tenderness, but if toxic megacolon occurs, perforation and peritonitis can result.

Pseudomembranous Enterocolitis

Pseudomembranous enterocolitis is an acute necrotizing slough of intestinal mucosa caused by overgrowth of the toxin-producing, gram-positive bacterium *Clostridium difficile*. Overgrowth occurs as a result of eradication of normal gastrointestinal flora by antibiotics. This adverse effect was originally associated with the use of clindamycin, but virtually every antibiotic has been implicated. The process may develop at any time during the course of antibiotic treatment, but usually occurs 5 to 7 days after initiation of treatment. There is no dose-response relationship; the condition has been reported after a single dose of antibiotics. Clinically, the patients develop abdominal distention, diffuse crampy pain, and diarrhea, which can occasionally be bloody. There may be associated high fever, tachycardia, and dehydration from the diarrhea. Endoscopy of the colon usually reveals the classic pseudomembranes or yellow-white, gray, or green, raised, exudative plaques. Ultimately the diagnosis is confirmed by detection of the clostridium toxin in the stool.

Allergies

Abdominal pain may result from primary or secondary involvement of the gastrointestinal tract in a patient having a major allergic reaction. In such cases the pain is intermittent but severe. During the acute phase of the allergic response, serous, watery fluid is secreted into the abdominal cavity. This results in distention with diffuse tenderness. The onset of such an attack may be rapid and resemble a strangulated intestine, pancreatitis, appendicitis, or ruptured ectopic pregnancy.

Constipation

Constipation may be a cause for abdominal pain and distention. Associated findings may include nausea, vomiting, and a low-grade fever. Spasms may be intense and mimic small-intestinal obstruction. Rectal examination and a plain roentgenogram of the abdomen should secure the diagnosis.

Irritable Bowel Syndrome

Irritable bowel syndrome may produce abdominal pain. The syndrome is often accompanied by distention and abnormal bowel habits, which are believed to be due to a disturbance of gastrointestinal motility.

Cystic Fibrosis

Cystic fibrosis (CF) in children may present with abdominal pain. Acute pancreatitis may be evident clinically and biochemically. Contrary to belief, children with CF and pancreatitis often have no endocrine or exocrine insufficiency. The pathophysiology is believed to be secondary to hyperconcentration of pancreatic secretions, which then leads to the acute inflammation. Children with idiopathic pancreatitis should have CF excluded as the underlying cause.

Organomegaly

Organomegaly, such as an enlarged spleen or liver, noted in a variety of disease entities (such as infectious mononucleosis or leukemia) will produce abdominal pain. Distention of Glisson's capsule probably explains pain associated with hepatomegaly. Massively enlarged spleens will often impinge on surrounding viscera and produce abdominal discomfort or early satiety. Once it is realized that the enlarged organ is the cause of the pain, the major task becomes to identify the cause of the enlargement.

Adhesions

Adhesions are a common cause of acute intestinal obstruction. Whether, in the absence of obstruction, adhesions can be the sole source of otherwise unexplained abdominal pain remains controversial. An occasional patient with chronic abdominal complaints undergoes an extensive diagnostic evaluation, culminating in a laparotomy or laparoscopy, during which adhesions are lysed and announced to be the cause of the pain. The patient, seemingly relieved, may even feel his or her condition improve temporarily. No scientific body of information, however, has conclusively implicated adhesions alone as a source of abdominal pain.

HEMATOPOIETIC SYSTEM

Lymphoma

Lymphoma may cause abdominal pain because of involvement of the spleen, the intestine itself, or the mesenteric or retroperitoneal nodes. The pain is rarely of a such a severe nature as to be confused with an acute abdomen. On occasion, however, a patient will present with acute intestinal obstruction secondary to involvement of the intestine or mesentary. Usually the patient has had a chronic problem with associated weight loss and night sweats.

Acute Leukemia

Acute leukemia may produce abdominal pain secondary to rapid enlargement of the spleen. Acute splenic infarction with intense, severe pain in the left upper quadrant accompanied by tenderness and muscular rigidity is an occasional complication.

Rupture of the Spleen

Splenic rupture from trauma or as a complication of infectious mononucleosis, malaria, or typhoid fever may occasionally occur. While this is generally a surgical problem, there is growing successful experience with nonoperative management. There is usually a history of trauma, even with a pathologic spleen, since spontaneous rupture is quite uncommon. The event may seem trivial, such as falling off a bicycle, or be unremembered during an episode of inebriation. Pain in the left upper quadrant or epigastrium predominates. Characteristically, diffuse, moderately severe pain with tenderness may occur from the irritating aspect of blood on the peritoneal surface. Kehr's sign (pain referred to either shoulder from diaphragmatic irritation) may be noted. Alternatively, the findings of the abdominal examination may be normal and a falling hematocrit level noted. The diagnosis is suspected based on history and a bloody peritoneal lavage or appropriate findings on computed tomography (CT).

Sickle-Cell Disease

The hemolytic crises of sickle-cell disease can result in fever, chills, abdominal pain, and backache. The sickled cells promote multiple intravascular thrombi, resulting in small infarcts in the spleen and other organs. Physical examination reveals moderate jaundice. The abdominal pain tends to be diffuse and of sudden onset, with occasional rebound tenderness, although this tends to improve rather quickly (24 to 48 hours) with hydration and exchange transfusion. When it does not respond, the physician should be suspicious of some precipitating event, like appendicitis or cholecystitis. The patient may note a subtle difference from the usual crisis pain; this should not be discounted. Laboratory data reveal anemia, reticulocytosis, and elevated levels of lactate dehydrogenase and total bilirubin. Acute hepatic sequestration mimicking cholecystitis or cholangitis can produce a diagnostic dilemma, since virtually all these patients also have cholelithiasis. Typically, with hepatic sequestration the alkaline phosphatase level is only minimally elevated, whereas with obstructive jaundice this canalicular enzyme is markedly increased.

Hemolytic Uremic Syndrome

The hemolytic uremic syndrome occurs during infancy and childhood and is characterized by abdominal pain, progressive renal failure, and a microangiopathic hemolytic anemia with thrombocytopenia. The colicky abdominal pain with associated nausea and vomiting may precede the hemolysis and renal failure by several days. Diarrhea and bloody stools may be noted and give the illusion of intussusception or ulcerative colitis. Intestinal infarction and perforation or intestinal ischemia with colonic strictures have all been reported. High temperatures (over 38°C) and marked leukocytosis (range, 20,000 to 50,000) with a left shift are not uncommon. The degree of leukocytosis does not correlate with the severity of the disease. There is oliguria or anuria with a concommitant rise in the serum blood urea nitrogen (BUN) and creatinine and the need for dialysis occasionally. Hypertension and cerebral involvement are prominent features. The mainstay of treatment is supportive.

Coagulation Disorders

Coagulation disorders, both hereditary and acquired, can lead to bleeding. Whether the blood loss occurs into the peritoneum or its contained structures or the retroperitoneum, abdominal pain can be a prominent manifestation. In hemophiliacs, spontaneous bleeding is common. Pseudoappendicitis has been reported when an intestinal wall hematoma presented with RLQ tenderness and guarding. Retroperitoneal hemorrhage can produce an ileus, with abdominal distention, vomiting, and a radiographic picture of an intestinal obstruction. Any patient on anticoagulants or with a history of a coagulopathy should have bleeding excluded prior to surgical intervention.

NEUROMUSCULAR AND SKELETAL DISORDERS

Herpes Zoster

Herpes zoster in an abdominal distribution may give rise to severe burning pain, which radiates in streaks from the back toward the middle of the abdomen. Characteristically, the pain does not cross the midline. Usually only one nerve segment is involved and there is localized pain. Although the burning, bandlike character of the pain is an important clue to the diagnosis, herpes zoster can be confused with biliary disease, renal colic, or appendicitis before the skin eruption occurs. As soon as the exanthem appears over the painful region, the diagnosis is easy. Of note, the pain occurs 2 to 4 days prior to the skin involvement.

Herniation of a Nucleus Pulposis

Herniation of a nucleus pulposus (lumbar disk) can occur suddenly and cause severe abdominal pain with radiation down the legs. Other causes of thoracolumbar pain that may be perceived as anterior abdominal in location include osteoarthritis, locked facets, spinal stenosis, or osteomyelitis.

Neoplasms of the Spinal Cord

Spinal cord neoplasms or space-occupying lesions (subarachnoid cyst) may, rarely, present with abdominal pain without associated gastrointestinal complaints. The abdominal pain may be diffuse or localized, but guarding is usually absent. Often the complaints are chronic and have been evaluated extensively. A thorough neurologic examination may reveal subtle hyperesthesias, weakness of the lower extremities, or pain with straight leg raises.

Nerve Entrapment Syndrome

Nerve entrapment syndrome may occur especially after a previous abdominal operation. Common locations are the ilioinguinal, iliohypogastric, genitofemoral, and rectus nerve distributions. The trapped nerve often produces exquisite, superficial tenderness over the involved area. Light palpation often causes the patient's eyes to tear, and there is excessive voluntary guarding and hysteric gyrations. The hover sign may be positive. To elicit this sign, the examiner simply places a hand over the area in question without touching the patient. The sign is positive if the patient squirms and grimaces. Extensive diagnostic investigations may produce normal findings, leading some clinicians to diagnose hysteria. However, injecting local anesthetic in the region of pain may alleviate the pain, confirming the diagnosis of entrapment.

Periostitis Pubis

Periostitis pubis is the term applied to chronic lower abdominal pain caused by inflammation of the pubic bone. The location of the problem is the site of insertion of the anterior abdominal musculature. It may be caused by an ill-placed suture during a herniorrhaphy. A physical examination reveals exquisite tenderness directly over the pubic tubercle. The laboratory findings are usually normal. Improvement occurs with local injection of a steroid.

Hernias of the Abdominal Wall

Hernias of the abdominal wall can produce abdominal pain and should be easily detected in the inguinal region. Spigelian or femoral hernias, however, have been overlooked. Likewise, a small primary hernia of the linea alba may go unnoticed and be the source of the pain. A thorough physical examination does not detect some of these hernias. When localized abdominal pain persists in the absence of a palpable mass, especially along the linea alba or semi-lunaris, ultrasonography or CT may reveal the hernia.

Spider Bites

Bites by a black widow (*Latrodectus mactans*) or a brown recluse (*Loxosceles reclusa*) spider may be associated with acute abdominal symptoms. The site of envenomation from both of these spiders initially reveals a modest in-flammatory response. Shortly afterward, the patient may experience malaise, dizziness, nausea, vomiting, and diffuse abdominal pain. Abdominal symptoms are usually mild after a recluse bite, whereas a lesion resembling pyo-derma gangrenosum may complicate the bite site. After a black widow bite a syndrome of lactrodectism may occur. This may be characterized by restless-ness, profuse perspiration, severe abdominal pain with boardlike rigidity, muscle twitching, gastric dilatation, ileus, and, rarely, death (less than 4%). Unless there is a known history of a bite, the diagnosis can be difficult.

METABOLIC AND ENDOCRINE DISEASES

Diabetic Ketoacidosis

Diabetic ketoacidosis (DKA) may be associated with abdominal pain, diffuse tenderness with muscular rigidity, and signs of peritonitis. If the patient is a known diabetic, the diagnosis can be suspected. In the absence of known dia-betes, the urinalysis is a good screening test, since it will reveal glucose and ketones. After hydration and treatment of DKA, most abdominal symptoms resolve quickly if they are of a nonsurgical nature. Of importance to note, how-ever, is that DKA can be precipitated by an underlying occult inflammatory process. Therefore, it is important to detect the acute appendicitis, cholecysti-tis, or perirectal abscess that may be the mechanism behind the DKA state. In addition, a diabetic neuropathy may involve the abdominal wall with resul-tant exquisite, superficial pain. An electromyogram can aid in this diagnosis.

Lead Poisoning

Lead poisoning in children still remains a major health problem in some large cities. It causes colicky abdominal pain accompanied by neurologic symp-toms (wrist drop, encephalopathy). The abdomen remains soft and non-tender. Blue lead lines may be seen in the patient's gingiva and the red blood cells show basophilic stippling.

Adrenal Insufficiency

Adrenal insufficiency (Addison's disease) can occur in a patient who was weaned too rapidly from steroid treatment or in a stressed patient with adrenal suppression from long-standing steroid usage. The syndrome produces fever, severe intermittent pain in the abdomen, continuous vomiting, and sometimes diarrhea. The pain continues as the patient rapidly deteriorates, shock being the most obvious finding. No localizing tenderness or involuntary guarding is noted. The serum sodium level tends to be high, with a low potassium. After adequate treatment with adrenal cortical hormones, pain completely and rapidly subsides.

Acute Porphyria
Acute porphyria can give rise to severe crampy abdominal pain, which is usually intermittent or recurrent. The pain, projectile vomiting, and distention most closely resemble a mechanical small-intestinal obstruction. As a rule, pain migrates from one side of the abdomen to the other without localizing signs. Patients may display rebound or rigidity, raising the concern for peritonitis. Often an abdominal scar from a previous, unrewarding laparotomy is noted. The subjective symptoms are usually judged to be exaggerated as compared with the objective findings, and the patient is easily labeled as hysterical. The symptoms are worsened by administration of barbiturates or sulfonamides. Porphyrins may characteristically be found in the urine, which becomes dark-red after exposure to light or upon standing for a period of time.

Hyperparathyroidism
Primary hyperparathyroidism is called "the disease of stones, bones, abdominal moans, and psychic overtones." The abdominal symptoms tend to be vague and nonspecific. Patients will complain of constipation and distention. The abdominal examination reveals only mild diffuse tenderness, without localizing signs or rebound. Pancreatitis occurs more commonly in patients with hyperparathyroidism, and therefore a calcium level should be obtained after the pancreatitis is resolved.

Familial Mediterranean Fever
Patients with familial Mediterranean fever have recurring abdominal pain that lasts 1 to 3 days every few weeks or months. Most patients are young, between 5 and 15 years old. There is usually a marked elevation in temperature, with associated tachycardia, malaise, and myalgias. Nausea and vomiting figure prominently in the symptoms. The pain may start in one area and spread throughout the entire abdomen. The abdomen is diffusely tender, with rebound pain. Leukocytosis can range from 15 000 to 30 000. The diagnosis can be very difficult, especially with a first attack.

Thyrotoxicosis
Thyroid storm (thyrotoxicosis) has been reported to present with abdominal pain, nausea, and vomiting. Diarrhea may also be noted from small- or large-intestine hypermotility. Associated symptoms include weight loss, fever,

tachycardia, chills, night sweats, and amenorrhea. The abdominal pain may be diffuse or localized, with guarding and rebound. The exact cause of the pain has not been elucidated. While abdominal complaints may predominate, the chief complaint, a thorough history, and physical examination should uncover the true diagnosis.

Electrolyte Depletion

Abdominal cramps may occur as a result of electrolyte depletion after excessive sweating. This is usually due to excess sodium and potassium loss. It has been noted in long distance runners, tri-athletes, and people who live in or visit tropical areas.

Hereditary Angioneurotic Edema

Hereditary angioneurotic edema (C1 esterase inhibitor deficiency) may cause abdominal pain. Patients usually have recurring bouts of swelling of the hands, face, and feet. It is an autosomal dominant, inheritable trait; therefore, a family history should be sought. Abdominal pain, while uncommon, can be associated with vomiting and tenderness. Attacks are usually self limiting and resolve in 24 to 72 hours.

Hyperlipoproteinemia

Hyperlipoproteinemia types I and V have been implicated in the precipitation of acute pancreatitis. In addition, hyperlipemic abdominal crises may cause recurrent, moderately severe abdominal pain not associated with pancreatitis. The etiology for this pain is unknown. Associated guarding and rigidity are demonstrable. The syndrome may be more common in younger women. Triglyceride levels during these attacks can range from 2000 to 6000 mg/dL. Generally, the pain will improve with intravenous fluids and cessation of oral intake. Control of the triglyceride levels will diminish the attacks.

Withdrawal from Drugs

Drug addiction withdrawal, such as with heroin, may be associated with abdominal symptoms and radiographic features of obstruction. Withdrawal symptoms usually include excessive perspiration, pale skin, "goose bumps," and dilated pupils, along with nervousness and hyperactivity. The patients may complain of leg cramps, and muscle twitching may be noted. Intestinal symptoms may be very acute during withdrawal and include vomiting, severe crampy abdominal pain, and diarrhea. Abdominal distention and distended small intestine may be noted on roentgenogram. The patient's complaints may be difficult to interpret, since they often exaggerate their symptoms in the hope of receiving narcotics. Therefore, differentiation among malingering, true abdominal pain, and the withdrawal syndrome may be challenging.

INFECTIOUS DISEASES

Malaria

Malaria, while not endemic in the United States, may still be seen occasionally, as a result of the ease of foreign travel. Cyclical chills, fever, and sweating are the classic symptoms; however, abdominal pain may also be prominent, especially in *Plasmodium falciparum* malaria. The abdominal pain is colicky, located in the midepigastrium, with little radiation. Backache may be noted separately. Nausea, vomiting, and diarrhea may accompany the abdominal pain. Hematochezia may occur as a result of intestinal ulcers. No real abdominal tenderness or rigidity is found on palpation of the abdomen, however. The spleen may be enlarged. Diagnosis is made by identification of the parasite in the peripheral blood smear approximately 6 hours after a chill.

Tuberculosis

Tuberculosis (TB) can produce abdominal pain by a variety of mechanisms. Tuberculosis of the spine may cause chronic back pain exacerbated by coughing or sneezing and perceived as abdominal in location. Tuberculous pleuritis may produce pain in the upper quadrants of the abdomen, depending on the amount of diaphragmatic and lower pleural involvement. Abdominal involvement with TB occurs when active pulmonary infection exists and swallowed sputa causes secondary tuberculous enteritis. This usually localizes in the ileocecal region and produces symptoms resembling appendicitis. Primary tuberculous peritonitis may occur, although the route of infection is not always clear and the symptoms may be very confusing. The classic "doughy abdomen" is seen only rarely. More typically the patient develops fever, ascites, inanition, and a tender mass in the lower abdomen. The pain is moderately severe, diffuse in location, and constant. Diarrhea may be prominent with ileal or colonic involvement. The diagnosis can be made by identification of acid-fast organisms from paracentesis fluid or by the appearance of multiple granulomas and adhesions at laparoscopy or laparotomy. Loops of intestine tend to be matted together and may obstruct.

Typhoid

Typhoid is sporadically found and occurs as a result of fecal contamination of food; it must be considered in the differential diagnosis of abdominal pain with fever. Mild, diffuse abdominal pain may develop over the course of 2 weeks, with moderate to severe pain during the peak of the illness. Nausea, vomiting, abdominal distention, and constipation may be the prodrome to the pain. Diarrhea then develops, followed by high fever, stupor, and delirium. *Salmonella typhi* can be cultured from the blood and stool.

Syphilis

Syphilis can involve every organ of the body, but abdominal involvement is usually a manifestation of tertiary syphilis or neurosyphilis. It will present as episodes of severe, acute, colicky abdominal pain (intestinal crises). When epigastric and continuous (gastric crisis), it may mimic a perforating ulcer. Retching and vomiting may be intense with the gastric crisis. Objective physical examination of the abdomen is normal; there is no involuntary muscular rigidity or rebound and the bowel sounds are normal. If the pupil responds to accommodation but not to light (Argyll Robertson pupil), tertiary syphilis is suspected and confirmed with appropriate blood tests.

Peritonitis

Primary peritonitis, a bacterial infection of the peritoneum without any identifiable intra-abdominal source, is occasionally seen in patients with cirrhosis, nephrosis, and ulcerative colitis. In children, the principal organism is the pneumococcus or hemolytic streptococcus; in adults coliforms predominate. The patients usually have ascites, but not always. Classic peritoneal signs are demonstrated on physical examination along with fever, vomiting, and diarrhea. On occasion laparotomy or laparoscopy will be necessary to exclude a surgically correctable problem.

Hepatitis

Hepatitis may produce mild to moderate abdominal distress because of inflammation and rapid enlargement of the liver. Tenderness is noted most prominently along the liver edge extending to the epigastrium and left upper quadrant, mimicking biliary colic. With acute cholecystitis there is more localized tenderness in the RUQ, rather than along the entire liver edge. Patients may complain of nausea and anorexia. A peculiar loss of the desire to smoke cigarettes has been noted. Levels of transaminases are usually elevated out of proportion to those of alkaline phosphatase, which leads one to the diagnosis.

Trichinosis

Trichinosis results from the ingestion of inadequately cooked pork containing the trichina worm. The patients may present with fever, myalgias, and edema, but colicky, periumbilical, moderately severe abdominal pain may also be noted. Nausea and vomiting may be prominent, but abdominal tenderness is minimal. The myalgias and edema are the key to the diagnosis, along with the history of pork ingestion. Eosinophilia may be noted in the differential blood count.

Amebiasis

Amebiasis is a parasitic disease infecting primarily the colon or liver, contracted through the ingestion of the cysts of *Entamoeba histolytica*. The clinical manifestations depend on the site of involvement. With colonic involvement, loose, watery, and even bloody diarrhea may predominate but can alternate with bouts of constipation. Fever and abdominal pain are variable. Amebic colitis may be confused with inflammatory bowel disease. Colonic perforation is a well-described phenomenon and generally presents with an acute abdomen. With localized cecal involvement (ameboma), the infection may simulate appendicitis. If a liver abscess exists, the pain may be continuous and localized to the right upper quadrant and radiate to the right shoulder. Hepatomegaly with point tenderness may be detected. Only a minority of patients with liver involvement will have active intestinal disease. Definitive diagnosis is made when the motile trophozoite is identified in the stool or a positive complement fixation test is obtained, suggesting liver involvement.

Ascariasis

Ascariasis may produce nonspecific abdominal complaints. Nausea, anorexia, and diarrhea predominate, but signs and symptoms of obstruction may occur. Abdominal tenderness, distention, and rebound pain mimicking an acute abdomen have been reported. The complete blood count may show eosinophilia. If obstruction exists, an abdominal plain roentgenogram may reveal a tangled mass of worms. This is evidenced by nearly parallel radiotranslucent lines from gas on top of the worms.

Rheumatic Fever

Rheumatic fever does not commonly have associated abdominal findings, but the pericarditis may produce epigastric discomfort. Associated heart failure may produce passive congestion of the liver and RUQ abdominal pain and tenderness. Abdominal distention, rebound, and rigidity are notably absent. Most patients will have a migratory polyarthritis, which should be a clue to the correct diagnosis. A cardiac murmur is sometimes detected.

Whipple's Disease

Whipple's disease is an uncommon generalized illness that produces a vague abdominal bloating, especially after meals. The cause is considered to be infectious because of the presence of a bacterial organism noted on electron microscopy of biopsied material. The pain, which is intermittent and periumbilical in location, is often accompanied by diarrhea. Anorexia and vomiting also are prominent in the symptoms. The abdomen reveals diffuse tenderness, almost a doughy consistency, with the suggestion of masses. A malabsorption syndrome is prominent, with progressive wasting. The diagnosis can be made by biopsy of a mesenteric node or biopsy of the small-intestinal mucosa.

Rocky Mountain Spotted Fever

Rocky Mountain spotted fever is an acute febrile illness associated with headaches, petechial rash, and occasional abdominal pain. The vector is the wood tick and the causative agent is *Rickettsia ricketsii.* The abdominal pain and tenderness may be localized and associated with rigidity as in acute appendicitis. Diarrhea and vomiting may be prominent in children. The tick bite may go unnoticed; however, recent travel in forested areas should raise suspicion.

Fitz-Hugh-Curtis Syndrome

Fitz-Hugh-Curtis syndrome is a periphepatitis associated with salpingitis. It is characterized by RUQ abdominal pain caused by inflammatory adhesions between the abdominal wall and the liver. The pain is pleuritic in nature and often exacerbated by coughing, breathing, or laughing. While antibiotic therapy is the prime treatment, laparoscopic lysis of adhesions is occasionally necessary.

SUGGESTED READING

Davis AE, Bradford WD. Abdominal pain resembling acute appendicitis in Rocky Mountain spotted fever. *JAMA*. 1982; 247:2811–2812.

Hershfield NB. The abdominal wall: a frequently overlooked source of abdominal pain. *J Clin Gastroenterol*. 1992; 14:199–202.

Jun PL, Slot H, Roos C. The acute abdomen in heroin addiction. *Br J Surg*. 1982; 69:598.

Katz S, Borst M, Seekri I, et al. Surgical evaluation of Henoch-Schönlein purpura: experience with 110 children. *Arch Surg*. 1991; 126:849–854.

Marenah CB, Quiney JR. C-1 esterase inhibitor deficiency as a cause of abdominal pain. *Br Med J*. 1983; 286:786.

McCoy HE, Kitchens CS. Small bowel hematoma in a hemophiliac as a cause of pseudoappendicitis: diagnosis by CT imaging. *Am J Hematol*. 1991; 38:138–139.

Miller A, Lees RS, McCluskey MA, et al. The natural history and surgical significance of hyperlipemic abdominal crisis. *Ann Surg*. 1979; 190:401–408.

Sawyers JL, Williams LF, eds. The acute abdomen. *Surg Clin North Am*. 1988; 68.

Snapper I. Extra-abdominal causes for abdominal pain. *Am J Gastroenterol*. 1982; 77:795–797.

CHAPTER 17

■

Clinical Management of Abdominal Pain When the Diagnosis Is in Doubt

Robert E. Condon, MD

PRINCIPLES

Not infrequently in a patient complaining of abdominal pain, no reasonably certain diagnosis can be made after eliciting a complete history, repeated physical examinations, and obtaining initial laboratory tests. In this distressing situation, a few principles should be kept in mind:

1. There are only a few diagnostic entities that may be made worse by abdominal exploration.
2. You can't make a diagnosis if you don't think of it.
3. Common things are common.

Only a Few Diseases Are Worsened by Laparotomy

In treating a patient with pain in the abdomen but in whom the diagnosis is in doubt, with few exceptions the safest course is to explore the abdomen if the signs and symptoms are compatible with peritonitis, viscus infarction, or intra-abdominal hemorrhage and are persisting or progressing. As far as possible, diseases that do not necessarily require laparotomy for treatment and that may be made worse by anesthesia and laparotomy should be excluded by appropriate examinations and tests. Among the conditions that may mimic an acute abdomen and be made worse by laparotomy are pneumonia, myocardial infarction, diabetic acidosis, acute hepatitis, pulmonary embolus, and severe heart failure (see Chapter 16).

To Make a Diagnosis, You Have to Think of It

This principle seems intuitively obvious, but in clinical situations it is commonly ignored. To help readers recall the possibility of various diagnoses associated with abdominal pain, some of which need a laparotomy for therapy but some of which do not, alternative diagnoses for patients complaining of right lower quadrant pain suggestive of appendicitis are displayed in Table 15. Possible diagnoses in patients complaining of more diffuse abdominal pain, in whom pain may originate from an extra-abdominal source, are reviewed in Chapter 16. In managing those patients with abdominal pain in whom the diagnosis seems obscure after initial evaluation, a glance through these lists of diagnostic possibilities often will help to focus further diagnostic efforts.

Common Things Are Common

Sometimes this is expressed as "when you hear hoofbeats don't think of zebras!" The reality, even when the diagnosis is in doubt, is that the more common causes of an acute abdomen are more likely to be the explanation for the symptoms than a rare or esoteric entity. Although the esoteric metabolic disorders are thought of first by the inexperienced, diseases of the genital, respiratory, cardiovascular, and urinary systems are far more common and more likely to cause or mimic an acute abdomen. Even when the cause of abdominal pain lies in an extraperitoneal organ, the principle applies.

TABLE 15. DISEASES CAUSING SYMPTOMS SUGGESTIVE OF APPENDICITIS

Pelvic inflammatory disease, including tubo-ovarian abscess (pyosalpinx)
Ectopic pregnancy
Ruptured graafian follicle
Ovarian cyst, twisted or not
Mesenteric adenitis
Yersinosis and other forms of enterocolitis
Acute ileitis (regional enteritis)
Intestinal tuberculosis
Lymphoma
Meckel's diverticulitis
Cecal diverticulitis
Sigmoid diverticulitis
Carcinoid tumor of the small intestine
Ruptured or expanding iliac aneurysm
Pancreatitis, especially with involvement of the right gutter
Perforating duodenal ulcer, especially with drainage into the right gutter
Acute cholecystitis

In nearly every patient with acute abdominal pain in whom the diagnosis is not obvious but in whom symptoms persist or progress, the surgeon should rule out as far as possible entities that may be worsened by laparotomy, briefly consider the possibilities of the less common diagnostic entities, and then explore the patient in the expectation that the cause most likely will be a common entity having an uncommon presentation.

OBSERVATION

Remember, the surgeon's primary goal is to avoid the development of diffuse peritonitis and shock. Usually, patients with definite and progressive acute abdominal signs and symptoms and who are at acceptable operative risk should have an exploratory laparotomy to establish the diagnosis and allow definitive treatment. But if the development and progression of the disease are slower, watchful waiting can sometimes be safer than an immediate operation. The surgeon must weigh all the factors in each case before deciding whether to operate or to wait. The criteria for exploratory laparotomy must be stricter when cardiac, vascular, pulmonary, or metabolic diseases are present and increase the patient's operative risk.

Observation of the abdomen requires repeated examinations at short intervals by the same examiner. Every patient with undiagnosed pain in the abdomen who does not require immediate operation must receive repeated clinical examinations. It is no disgrace to be unsure after only one examination, but it is wrong to rely on only one examination when an obscure abdominal process exists. Repeated examination by the same examiner is the way to avoid mistakes.

Recording pulse and temperature changes is more helpful in slowly progressing obscure situations than in a more acute abdomen. Laboratory and roentgenographic examinations should be repeated as indicated, but the main emphasis must be on clinical examination of the patient. Observation of the abdomen should not cease until a diagnosis is made, an exploratory laparotomy is decided upon, or the risk of peritonitis or hemorrhage subsides.

This evaluation of the patient and his or her disease is the surgeon's responsibility. *The decision to operate or not cannot be undertaken by or delegated to any other physician.*

LAPAROSCOPY

In some patients, the initial exploration is carried out laparoscopically. The diagnostic utility of laparoscopy has been somewhat overlooked, but it is a very efficient method to establish a diagnosis or to rule out involvement of most of the abdominal and pelvic viscera. Only the retroperitoneal organs are inadequately visualized, but secondary signs of retroperitoneal disease may be discernible. In some instances, eg, acute appendicitis, laparoscopy provides not only a means to establish a diagnosis but also can be a therapeutic modality.

EXPLORATORY LAPAROTOMY

An exploratory laparotomy is indicated when a disease causing peritonitis or intra-abdominal hemorrhage is suspected and the suspicion cannot be eliminated. The operation should not be begun until hemoconcentration, anemia, oliguria, acidosis, and hyperthermia have been corrected. Shock must be treated first, especially in children and in advanced cases of peritonitis.

When the abdomen is opened, the peritoneum is carefully observed for reddening and edema. The amount and appearance of peritoneal fluid are observed. Is the fluid clear and serous? Cloudy or purulent? Sanguinous or bloody?

Clear, Serous Peritoneal Fluid

If the peritoneal exudate is clear and serous, look at the appendix first. Next examine the small intestine for the presence of a Meckel's diverticulum, enlarged lymph glands in the mesentery, signs of enteritis, or obstruction. After examining the small intestine, the genital organs should be palpated and the pelvic peritoneum examined. The ovaries and tubes are drawn out through the incision and inspected for salpingitis, follicular rupture, or twisting of cysts. The sigmoid colon is examined next for diverticulitis or tumor, and then the rest of the colon is methodically examined. The gallbladder is palpated, feeling for stones and degree of distention. The pancreas is palpated and inspected for scarring, swelling, or hemorrhage. The stomach and duodenum are next examined for ulceration or tumor. Samples of fluid from the upper portion of the abdominal cavity can, as a rule, be obtained at this time. Before the abdomen is closed, the following diseases must be excluded:

- appendicitis
- Meckel's diverticulitis
- regional enteritis
- perforated intestine
- intestinal infarction
- intestinal obstruction
- salpingitis and pelvic inflammatory disease
- ectopic pregnancy
- twisted ovarian cyst
- ruptured ovarian follicle (Mittelschmerz)
- acute cholecystitis

- acute pancreatitis
- perforating duodenal or gastric ulcer or tumor
- acute diverticulitis

Cloudy or Purulent Fluid

If the peritoneal exudate is purulent or appears so, peritonitis exists and its cause must be traced. A sample from the peritoneum should be taken for Gram's stain, smear, and culture. Appearances can be deceiving. Turbid to opaque, fibrinous, thin fluid may actually be pus resulting from bowel perforation or a similar cause of bacterial contamination. Purulent-appearing fluid, on the other hand, may contain no bacteria but may represent an abundant cellular response of the peritoneum to a sterile or nearly sterile irritant, as in perforating duodenal ulcer.

The appendix is examined first. If the appendix is normal, the small intestine should be examined from the ileocecal valve to the duodenal-jejunal flexure for Meckel's diverticulitis, perforation of the intestine by a foreign body, obstruction, ulceration, infarct with perforation, tumor, or enteritis. The omentum is pulled out to exclude the possibility of gangrenous or infarcted omentum. The large intestine is investigated for diverticulitis, cancer, obstruction, perforation, or infarct. The genitalia are palpated for salpingitis, infected genital tumor, or twisted cyst. The gallbladder is examined for stones and degree of distention and edema. The pancreas is palpated for swelling. The duodenal bulb and pylorus are examined for perforation.

If the cause of the peritonitis still cannot be definitely ascertained, an examination of the duodenum (using a Kocher maneuver) and of the ventral and dorsal sides of the stomach is made. This may require a new incision in the upper abdomen. If there is still no explanation for the peritonitis, the Gram's stain of the peritoneal exudate is examined to demonstrate a possible primary peritonitis (pneumococci, streptococci, *E coli*, tuberculosis). With the occurrence of cloudy exudate in the abdominal cavity at laparotomy, the cause of peritonitis must be determined with certainty before the abdomen is closed.

Sanguinous or Bloody Peritoneal Fluid

If the peritoneal exudate is sanguinous or bloody, the cause must always be demonstrated. Sanguinous (blood-tinged) exudate can be caused by:

- obstruction with distention
- intestinal infarction
- perforation of the intestine
- ruptured ectopic pregnancy
- rupture of ovarian follicle (Mittelschmerz)
- infarct in a solid abdominal organ
- necrotic pancreatitis
- trauma—blunt or penetrating—to the abdominal wall or to the viscera

Frank blood in the abdomen occurs with:

- ruptured spleen
- ruptured ectopic pregnancy
- ruptured liver
- ruptured aortic or mesenteric aneurysm
- ruptured kidney
- rupture of an abdominal tumor
- penetrating trauma to the abdominal wall or viscera

Exploratory laparotomy must determine and control the source of bleeding with certainty, and the operation must not be terminated before this certainty is obtained.

Index

Date Due

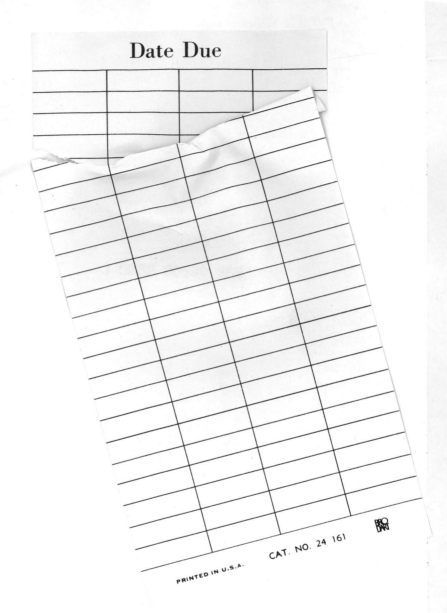

CAT. NO. 24 161

PRINTED IN U.S.A.